THE INTOLERANT
GOURMET

GLORIOUS FOOD WITHOUT GLUTEN & LACTOSE

BARBARA KAFKA

ARTISAN

ALSO BY BARBARA KAFKA

Vegetable Love

Soup: A Way of Life

Roasting: A Simple Art

Party Food

The Opinionated Palate

Microwave Gourmet Healthstyle Cookbook

Microwave Gourmet

Food for Friends

American Food and California Wine

Published by Artisan
A division of Workman Publishing
Company, Inc.
225 Varick Street
New York, NY 10014-4381
www.artisanbooks.com

Published simultaneously in Canada by
Thomas Allen & Son, Limited

Library of Congress
Cataloging-in-Publication Data

Kafka, Barbara.
The intolerant gourmet : glorious food
without gluten and lactose / Barbara Kafka.
p. cm.
Includes index.
ISBN 978-1-57965-394-1 (hardback)
1. Gluten-free diet—Recipes. 2. Wheat-free
diet—Recipes. 3. Milk-free diet—Recipes.
I. Title.
RM237.86.K34 2011
641.5'638—dc22
2011005683

Design by Kevin Brainard
Food styling by Christine Albano
Prop styling by Michelle Wong

Printed in China

First printing, October 2011

10 9 8 7 6 5 4 3 2 1

To all those who have helped me over the years, particularly Chris Styler and the late Kathi Long. And, with love, to those I acknowledge on page 233.

CONTENTS

BEFORE WE BEGIN

I and many others are Intolerant Gourmets, lovers of good food who are celiac, unable to digest gluten (wheat, oats, and barley), which is to be gluten intolerant. I also, like many, cannot tolerate the lactose of milk in any form. These are both genetic autoimmune diseases that are not always active in the person who has them. They are often activated—particularly in infants and small children—by eating the taboo foods. However, it has been discovered in recent years that the genes that cause these intolerances can be activated for no known reason, even quite late in life.

Many of us are intolerant of bad food, ersatz food, and poor cooking. Despite my problems and my character, I have found that I can cook excellent food and, on my way to this happy present, I have learned a great deal about the art, theory, and practice of using unfamiliar ingredients and making things that are delicious.

In childhood, I was conspicuous, being an outsider at birthday parties, unable to eat ice cream and cupcakes due to the inevitable gluten and lactose. I had these troubles, which my children later inherited. The symptoms of these intolerances seemed to go away as I got older—except for an unpleasant tendency to foul the air with gas.

Perhaps my passion for food was brought on by my early deprivation; but my literary ambitions and delight in making good things to please people grew into a way of life and finally a career. Cooking for one is not my pleasure—I don't normally cook for myself—but I adore making food for friends and gradually became a food writer and at one point even had a flourishing business as a consultant to restaurants, food stores, and food manufacturers. I wrote many books. Some of them were great, thick tomes. I wrote for magazines, newspapers, and almost everyone who asked. I spouted words on radio and television. It was hard work, but fun.

Then, as I got older, the old symptoms returned and I had to change what I cooked and avoid writing about many dishes, as I couldn't taste all things and I will not give a recipe for anything I cannot stand behind. I thought that I had reached an age at which to stop writing. However, good friends convinced me that what I was learning should be made into yet one more book, that it was a gift worth giving. Besides, I missed the act of writing and having contact with readers, cooks, and eaters. I didn't miss cooking and eating because they were constants in my life.

Writing this book is not just about me. For some reason that no one seems to understand, the number of the gluten intolerant has increased ten times in recent years. It has always been true that 60 percent of the population cannot fully digest dairy (lactose). Although they are unrelated genetically, lactose intolerance and gluten intolerance often occur in the same person. These intolerances are not allergies, but genetic disorders that make life difficult and unpleasant. They can vary in evidencing their presence or intensity over time; but they do not disappear. I must limit what I make and eat. No one for whom I cook seems to complain and I hope that by sharing what I do, I can make some lives a great deal more pleasant without a great deal of work.

NOT A PLAGUE: A BLESSING

Those of us who are Intolerant Gourmets—either of gluten, lactose, or both—tend to think that we have a disease and perhaps even a curse. In truth, while it is a disease and difficult to live with, it may be a blessing in disguise. Certainly it has been shown that simple, rapidly digested carbohydrates,

2

of which wheat flour is one, disrupt the normal digestion in ways other than the evident. Their rapid absorption into the system does funny things to insulin production and can lead the way to diabetes as well as other unpleasant things. All nutrition is more complicated than this; but it may give some comfort.

SENSATIONS PLUS TASTES

Food is not just about flavor. It is also about sensation. I think that the lavish usual usage of butter and cream provides silkiness while carrying flavors. Butter and cream are hard to replace; but as I have tested recipes and written this book, I am constantly endeavoring to find equivalent replacements for the pleasure. The natural gelatin from good stock or added commercial gelatin, egg yolks, coconut milk, and various oils from olive to toasted sesame all help in part. I have also found that certain nuts and legumes puréed help as well. I hope that soon the craving for lactose will leave you and the desire for silky sensation will be satisfied.

ALMOST EVERYTHING YOU WANT TO EAT

This is a book that will satisfy your need for mashed potatoes and other buttery dishes and pastas—but not with substitutes and eccentricities. It is meant to serve as an all-purpose cookbook for us intolerants and our intolerant friends and family. In many cases this has meant rethinking or reformulating classic recipes without the use of flour or butter as a thickener, or the use of butter as a base for cooking and cream to round out a sauce. There are, of course, really new recipes; I can never resist the lure of the kitchen.

I hope that I have written a book that will make it possible for all of us to enjoy these foods without

3

recourse to ersatz ingredients or expensive bought items often using a wide range of chemicals.

One of the few things that I serve that I don't make is pasta. There are companies that seem to have conquered the art of making pasta without using wheat flour. I have found only one brand of gluten-free bread that has been reasonable; the rest have invariably proved disappointing, and even the good one is best when toasted, since it's fragile.

SANDWICH GOOD-BYE

I think the hardest thing about going on a gluten-free diet was being deprived of sandwiches. I've never been much of a breakfast eater so it was only rarely that I coveted someone's crisp toast slathered in butter (whoops, lactose). What I missed most were very American things: a street-cart frankfurter, a tuna sandwich on toast with mayo, lettuce, and tomato, or a BLT—let alone a pastrami on rye. I mourned my favorite, the fully summer-ripe tomato, dripping into the kitchen-sink sandwich with mayo out of a jar on commercial, squooshy white bread.

I still haven't recovered. Yes, I've tried the valiant attempts at gluten-free bread—imagine my dismay when one of my favorite restaurants in Venice offered me gluten-free bread and after eating it (actually gorging on it), I became ill. A little reflection and a little research detected the ample presence of butter and milk. I have even come up with my own gluten-free white bread (delicious but too fragile for sandwiches, it makes great toast—see page 17); but this hasn't been the comfort that many of the gluten-free commercial pastas have. I did discover that I could make a reasonable imitation of a sandwich using corn tortillas heated up for about thirty seconds in the microwave.

A compensation has been the exciting discovery of grains that were unfamiliar to me although ancient in history. I have fallen in love with pre-rinsed quinoa, teff, and millet.

Additionally, I have turned to many Asian recipes since these cuisines generally do not use dairy products or wheat. I have made no attempt to pretend to be an Asian cook; instead, I have used these genres and their ingredients as inspirations.

I was never a pastry chef or a passionate baker; but restaurants and many friends crave these things. Hence I created a large group of recipes for sweet desserts. While I must admit that I get cranky in restaurants where servers apprised of my restrictions smilingly offer me a lovely sorbet, for this book I developed a group of sorbets that even please me, as well as special gluten- and lactose-free sweets.

The Intolerant Gourmet follows the usual order of cookbooks, except for the closing section that is all about the starches (flours, grains, pulses, beans, and seeds), as these are the most problematical (oil for butter is a cinch). That section has no recipes but contains all of the basic preparations. The recipes turn up in their normal place in the book.

One more note and confession: another book I've written, *Roasting: A Simple Art,* is ideal for people with my kind of restrictions. I cannot simply repeat large sections of that book; but I can recommend it. In this book, there are new recipes for roasting, not new techniques, but new foods that have never contained the taboo foods.

New or old I hope that readers will tolerate me and enjoy the food. They don't have to be Intolerant Gourmets to do so. This is food to be shared by all.

THE INTOLERANT GOURMET PANTRY

This is a list of some items that may not be on your shelves, but that I find make gluten- and dairy-free cooking and eating easier. There are obviously no wheat or wheat flour, oatmeal, and barley in the book and certainly no milk foods (lactose).

I assume that most of us have salt and pepper and other common seasonings and ingredients. Here I list only those items that may be new to the cook. It used to be hard to find many of them and it often meant a trip to a specialty shop. Many can be found in ordinary markets or online.

GRAINS: Amaranth, buckwheat, chestnut flour, corn (flour, masa harina, meal, polenta, starch, popcorn), garbanzo flour, potato starch, quinoa, rice bran, rice flour, tapioca flour, and teff (seeds and flour). See the entries in Stiff Upper Lip: The Starches (page 210) for more information.

PASTA, NOODLES, ETC.: Gluten-free pasta, rice (paper, wrapper, noodles, sticks), and mung bean noodles/threads. Gluten-free pasta can be bought and is satisfactory (see the chart on page 39). Rice and mung bean products are excellent gluten-free substitutes.

OILS, VINEGARS, AND CONDIMENTS: Harissa (a Moroccan spicy seasoning paste), rice vinegar (a mild vinegar less dominant than others), safflower oil (neutral in flavor and can be heated to very high heat), toasted sesame oil (chestnut brown in color, it has a warm, delicious flavor; it should not be confused with golden-colored plain sesame oil and it should not be overheated), sherry vinegar (brown in color, somewhat unusual and rich in flavor), and gluten-free soy sauce.

COCONUT MILK: While coconut milk has a flavor of its own, it can be substituted for regular milk in many recipes with appropriate seasonings. Take care; there are thick coconut milks. I use the ordinary kind, buying it in cans.

SEASONINGS: Anchovies (whole packed in oil and anchovy paste), black mustard seeds, caraway seeds, capers (packed in salt), chocolate (dark—no milk chocolate), espresso powder, fermented black beans (available at Asian grocery stores, these have a salty deep taste), dried mushrooms (shiitake; porcini, which give depth of flavor to ordinary mushrooms), ras el hanout (a spicy Arabic seasoning powder), sardines (whole packed in oil), star anise (an Asian spice with a faint licorice taste), and sumac (used in the Middle East, deep dark purple sumac grows on bushes).

Keep in mind that the more usual seasonings, seeds, and herbs (fresh and dried) can vary in flavor, often according to their place of origin. For instance, Syrian oregano is more pungent than Italian—or, for that matter, than what I grow myself. Spices also diminish in intensity with time.

READING LABELS

One of the most annoying things about being a gluten- and lactose-free cook is the need to read the tiny-type lists of ingredients. (It helps to bring reading glasses to the market.) Gluten and lactose can hide in the lists under semivisible names. Watch out for wheat starch, whey, and various other particles of wheat, oats, barley, and milk products including butter, sour cream, and cheese. Often packaged foods will contain taboo foods if not evidently. When in doubt, avoid them.

NO-NO AND TABOO

Wheat is still the chief culprit, but it is wise to know when reading labels or menus that it goes disguised by *many* names. I started a list because I was confused by a mention of corn gluten. Among the "hidden" names of wheat are bulgur or burghul, triticale (triticale is actually a mix with rye, as is mir), spelt (dinkle), and farro. More wheats: durum (Emmer), einkorn, farina (as in cereal), fu, kamut, matzo, milo, semolina, and Graham flour, as well as the self-evident wheat berry, wheat germ, wheat gluten, wheat nut, and wheat starch. Finally, there's seitan, which is often used in vegetarian dishes.

In addition, barley, rye, and oats should all be avoided.

Those wanting to know more about gluten intolerance can go to the website of the Celiac Sprue Association, www.csaceliacs .org/gluten_grains.php.

HOW WE DO IT

Like most crafts and arts do, cooking has a specialized language. The words in cooking are often derived from the French; some, like *purée* or *sauté,* more obviously than others. Many are not. They can be thought of as a shorthand describing a variety of techniques. This avoids repeating longer instructions. While this book cannot list all of them, I thought it might be helpful to give a selection of those terms that I use frequently.

DREDGING

To dredge something means to coat it evenly. It is usually followed by the word "in" and then some sort of dry ingredient, such as teff flour, cornstarch, or rice flour. Other times some sort of liquid used as a coating—egg yolks, egg wash, etc.—will be added to the process before the dry ingredients are put on.

Dredging is useful for two important reasons. First, it forms a protective coating that seals in moisture. Second, that coating browns well to form a golden crust when exposed to hot fat.

Items can be dredged in dry ingredients and then cooked in hot oil or can be dredged in a multistep process beginning and ending with dry ingredients with a dredging in liquid in between. The added liquid step creates a thicker, more insulating protective coating.

BOILING

Some of the most comforting meals for cold, bleak midwinter days are boiled treats—traditional one-pot meals with broth, meats, vegetables, and herbs. Unfortunately for time-pressed cooks, the recipes are throwbacks to the days when time was not in such short supply and the cost of ingredients was more of a concern.

But who has the luxury of time today? The only solution is to reformulate dishes like shabu-shabu—a fonduelike beef and vegetable dish from Japan by way of New England whose onomatopoeic name suggests the sound the meat makes as it goes into the broth—so that they can be completed more quickly. This requires some cleverly thought out shortcuts, some relatively expensive foods, and maybe even some tight-lipped secrecy around the stove. One does not have to admit to using prepared ingredients like canned stock.

Once the accelerating, expediting, and recipe rejiggering have been done, feasts such as Chinese Chicken in the Pot (page 88), Luxury Boiled Beef (page 105), and Apple-Cider-Rich Boiled Tongue Dinner (page 139) can be ready in about an hour. The best way to serve them is in big, old-fashioned rimmed soup dishes, accompanied by knives, forks, and large soupspoons. If the dishes are unavailable, serve the solids on dinner plates and give each person a bowl of soup on the side. In that case, the noodles or rice should go into the bowl.

A few terms:

Rolling boil: large bubbles form and continue to rise.

Medium boil: smaller bubbles form continuously.

Low boil: only occasional bubbles form.

Simmer: bubbles are mainly around the edge of the pot.

GRILLING AND BROILING

The main distinction between these two ways of cooking seems to be the outdoor macho associated with grilling. I would even argue that it was James Beard with his writing on grilling that made it all right for men to cook as a nonprofessional activity.

That was then. Today, many men cook to entertain or for pleasure.

There are, of course, other significant differences between the two modes. When grilling, the heat comes from beneath, and when broiling it usually comes from above. Always place the wire rack closest to the heat source. For oven broiling, place the rack on the top level of the oven. For grilling, place the rack low and close to the heat.

Come the warm days of summer, eating and entertaining outdoors is not only a possibility, but a pleasure. It may also be a necessity if your house is, like mine, at times swarmed by people who have come to swim or chat or stay.

Of course, these meals can be eaten indoors if the weather is too hot or buggy. In any case, such meals tend to be less formal than winter meals. People may even wander around with a glass in their hands.

Grilling is a good option, and I give several possibilities in my book *Party Food* in which I envisage eaters having their grilled food on grilled bread, or it can be roasted as in *Roasting: A Simple Art.*

It is hard to give precise instructions for grilling. The most important variable is the fire. Start it a good hour before it will be needed; alternatively, leave enough time so that the coals are white hot before you start cooking. How to heat the grill is also important to how food will taste. Mesquite, oak, charcoal, etc., add more tasty flavors to food than conventional gas.

Meat for grilling and broiling should be relatively tender, vegetables cut into broad strips, fruit left whole unless very large. Nothing should be too thick. Remember, the high heat will cook things quickly. All things to be cooked like this need a thin slick of oil all over them unless there is a marinade. Turn food fairly often and check for doneness.

Special tools are useful: tongs, sleeved pot holders, sturdy spatulas, and, for grilling, long-handled forks. Don't forget the grill brush to clean the grill off thoroughly for next time. While I have heard it said that leftover bits of food "add flavor," I think it's just an excuse not to clean.

TOLERANT ROASTING

I believe roasting is one of the best techniques for savory food without gluten or lactose. I've written a whole book on roasting, *Roasting: A Simple Art,* and I don't propose to rewrite it in this book, although I will give a few new recipes using my basic high-heat method. Open the window, turn on the exhaust, keep the oven clean, and if need be, remove the batteries from the smoke detectors. Put them back after eating. Except for the starches (but yes for potatoes), almost all of the normal foods in the meal or the kitchen can be roasted, from vegetables through fish, poultry, meat, and fruits.

Roasted food has a rich flavor, and in the case of meats the internal fats obviate the need for adding more.

DEGLAZING

Today, "no fat" is the name of the game. I must say that I am sometimes tempted to leave a little fat in the sauce for added unctuousness. To remove the fat before deglazing, transfer the main ingredients to a platter, tilt the roasting pan so that all the liquid collects in one corner, and pour off or spoon out excess fat. To deglaze, put the roasting pan, fresh from the oven (main ingredients transferred to a platter), on top of the stove. Add water, wine, or stock and boil while scraping the bottom vigorously with a wooden spoon. If not using a nonstick pan and the residue is particularly stubborn, use a metal spatula for scraping. Boil until the liquid is reduced by half.

Deglazing makes the base of a gravy. It also cleans the pan. Pour the gravy into a sauceboat or bowl or pour it over the cooked food.

THICKENING

Many sauces and stews need to be thickened toward the end of cooking. The most commonly used thickener—flour cooked in butter—is clearly no good for us. However, there are many alternatives. Some of the hot liquid can be stirred into lightly beaten egg yolks before being cooked in the dish. Dishes can also be thickened with puréed starches such as chickpeas.

A slurry is perhaps the best thickener for Intolerants. Arrowroot or cornstarch is mixed with a little cold water, and then with some of the hot liquid that is being thickened. It is then poured into the liquid needing thickening and then cooked—usually briefly.

BREAKFAST

I have never been a big breakfast eater. Most people seem to relish opening the day with something good, which is a problem for the gluten and lactose challenged since practically all typical breakfast foods contain gluten or lactose. Though there are now gluten-free cereals, they are less appealing when deprived of milk. While the following recipes will not assuage all breakfast longings, they should help. The recipe I developed for waffles is a triumph and a treat for both Intolerant Gourmets and their gluten- and dairy-loving friends. The meager selection of breads contains no odd chemicals and tastes good. Most of them should be toasted to be at their best. There is even a very good hot cereal.

Eggs, bacon, and ham as well as smoked fish are always a pleasure. Be careful of sausages. Many of them include some form of wheat as a filler. Fruits and juices are no problem. However, I have had to do some playing with hot chocolate to make it okay.

WAFFLES

These are so good that my husband ate the entire batch covered in maple syrup while I was out of the kitchen fixing my computer.

They are light and elegant and could equally well serve as a dessert if topped with Raspberry Sauce (page 199) or Chocolate Sauce (page 199). If your friends love these, make double or triple the dry ingredients and store until you're ready to make a batch.

It is true that the variety of flours may be new; but today most of them are available at markets, and in health-food stores or on the web. SEE COLOR PLATE 6

¼ cup tapioca flour

½ cup garbanzo bean (chickpea) flour

½ cup potato starch

¾ cup white rice flour

1 tablespoon baking powder

1 teaspoon kosher salt

2 cups coconut milk

2 eggs

½ cup plus 1 tablespoon safflower oil

Turn a waffle iron to high.

Mix the dry ingredients in a medium bowl. In another bowl, whisk the coconut milk, eggs, and ⅜ cup of the oil together. Then whisk the wet ingredients into the flour mixture until well combined.

Evenly brush both the top and bottom of the hot waffle iron with 1 to 2 teaspoons of the remaining oil. Pour ½ cup batter for each waffle (the iron we used makes two waffles at a time; if yours is much smaller, use ⅓ cup batter) and close the waffle iron. Cook for 5 to 6 minutes, or until the waffles are crisp and golden brown (the waffles are crisper when less oil is used to grease the waffle iron).

MAKES EIGHT 5-×-6-INCH WAFFLES

QUINOA HOT CEREAL

Breakfast can be a bit difficult for Intolerant Gourmets, but once again quinoa comes to the rescue. This is as good as any hot cereal on the market and is loaded with calcium to boot.

½ cup quinoa

2 tablespoons maple syrup

¼ teaspoon freshly grated nutmeg, plus some to sprinkle on top (optional)

Bring 2 cups water to a boil over high heat, pour in the quinoa, and then return to a boil. Cover and reduce the heat to a simmer. Cook for 45 minutes. Add the maple syrup and nutmeg and serve.

MAKES 2 CUPS

WHITE BREAD

This recipe would not be possible without the late Bette Hagman and her book *The Gluten-Free Gourmet Bakes Bread*. She was innovative and to be respected. I made a few changes to avoid artificial ingredients, but the credit is hers.

The bread also makes great toast.

French Meadow Bakery makes a similar good loaf, available online and in specialty stores.

½ cup tapioca flour

¾ cup garbanzo bean (chickpea) flour

1 cup potato starch

1¼ cups white rice flour

2½ teaspoons dry yeast

2 tablespoons sugar

1 tablespoon ground flax seeds

1½ teaspoons kosher salt

3 eggs

¼ cup plus 1½ teaspoons safflower oil

1½ cups warm water, or more if needed

Mix the dry ingredients in a large bowl until well combined. In another bowl, stir the eggs, ¼ cup of the oil, and the water together. Pour the wet ingredients into the dry ingredients and mix well by hand. The dough should look like cake batter; if it does not, add more warm water a tablespoon at a time until it does. Move the bowl to a warm place and let it sit for 1 hour.

With the rack in the middle of the oven, turn the heat to 400°F. Grease a 7½-×-3½-×-3-inch metal loaf pan with the remaining safflower oil. Pour the batter into the greased pan and bake for 50 to 55 minutes, covering the top of the bread lightly with aluminum foil after the first 10 minutes. Turn the loaf out onto a wire rack by carefully running a knife along the edges of the pan and inverting. Allow to cool before slicing.

MAKES 1 LOAF WITH SIXTEEN ½-INCH-THICK SLICES

AREPAS

Arepas are the pita breads of Colombia, Venezuela, and other parts of South America. They are made from corn and puff up nicely. They can be eaten as a bread or split open like a pita, stuffed, and rebaked. They are simple and a pleasure. They do not turn dark or form a crisp crust.

There are special pans for making them as well as mixes that can be found online.

Do not substitute another from of masa (see headnote, page 18).

2 cups masa harina

1½ teaspoons kosher salt

2 cups warm water

Combine the ingredients in a medium bowl. Knead well until the mixture is uniform and easy to handle; there will no longer be any dry spots nor will it be sticky. Cover with plastic wrap and set aside for 30 minutes.

Place a large nonstick sauté pan (about 12 inches across) over medium heat. Measure out the dough into ¾-cup balls and form into discs 3½ inches wide and ⅜ inch thick. Reduce the heat to low, place four discs in the pan, and cook for 15 to 20 minutes. Turn the discs over and cook another 15 to 20 minutes, until they are dry to the touch on both sides. Transfer to a platter to dry out completely for 45 minutes. Repeat for another batch. Enjoy immediately or keep in a tightly sealed plastic bag at room temperature for 4 to 5 days.

MAKES 8 AREPAS

NOTE

To Freeze Arepas

Separate the arepas with parchment or wax paper and store in a tightly sealed freezer bag for up to several weeks. Defrost each in a microwave oven for 1 minute.

ENGLISH MUFFINS

These really do look and taste like their gluten- and dairy-laden counterparts. Just don't expect quite as many nooks and crannies.

It is extremely important to use masa harina for this recipe. Though it is a corn product, it is completely different from cornmeal and masarepa (produced specifically for arepas although I still find that the masa harina arepas are much tastier). Masa harina is traditionally used to make corn tortillas and tamales but can make arepas as well (see the preceding recipe). The more coarsely ground cornmeal is used to make corn bread and corn mush.

1¼ cups masa harina
1¼ cups warm water
½ teaspoon kosher salt
Dough for ⅓ recipe White Bread (page 17)

Combine the masa harina, water, and salt and mix well. Cover with plastic wrap and set aside.

Allow the bread dough to rise in a warm place for an hour.

Mix the masa harina dough and the White Bread dough together by hand until uniform. Place a 10-inch nonstick skillet over medium heat. Scoop out ⅓ cup dough at a time and roll it into a 2-inch ball. Place 4 or 5 balls in the pan at a time (evenly spaced apart and not touching) and flatten slightly with the palm of your hand to form 3-inch discs. Cook for 5 to 7 minutes, then flip over with a spatula and cook for 5 to 6 minutes more, until dry to the touch on both sides.

MAKES 9 ENGLISH MUFFINS

EGGS FLORENTINE

This is a truly fantastic rendition of the original dish. Assembling all the different parts is a bit time consuming but well worth the effort. Enjoy alone or invite friends over for brunch.

2 tablespoons olive oil
2 bunches fresh spinach (about 6 ounces each), stemmed, washed well, and dried (about 8 cups)
Kosher salt
Freshly ground black pepper
2 English Muffins (preceding recipe)
4 Perfect Poached Eggs (page 19)
1 cup Basic Mayonnaise (page 190)
Pinch cayenne pepper

Place the oil in a 10-inch nonstick skillet over medium-high heat. When the oil shimmers, drop the spinach into the pan. Sauté the spinach until it is tender and dark green, 1 to 2 minutes. Season with salt and pepper to taste.

Cut in half and toast the English muffins. Put two halves on each plate. Place a quarter of the sautéed spinach on each muffin half. Put one poached egg on top of the spinach. Add the mayonnaise and 1 tablespoon water to a double boiler. Stir constantly just until the mayonnaise is warm (if it gets hot, it will separate). Season with cayenne. Pour a quarter of the sauce over each egg.

SERVES 2 WITH 2 EGGS EACH

PERFECT POACHED EGGS

When I first started to cook, I was terrified of poaching eggs because I had heard so many tales about how things could go wrong. Since I was following standard practices of the day, horrible results were almost inevitable.

For example, my first, scantily equipped kitchen came with an aluminum device with five circular depressions. You cracked eggs one by one into each hollow and then set the contrivance over boiling water. The resulting poached eggs were tough and ghastly.

A noted food writer suggested creating a series of whirlpools in a pot by vigorously stirring boiling water in a circle and then dropping an egg into the maelstrom. This risky undertaking was repeated for each egg in turn. Many attempts at this still left egg whites broken apart pathetically in the water.

The standard chefs' trick is to add vinegar to the cooking water. This does help congeal the whites, but all the rinsing in the world does not eliminate the vinegar taste.

Happily, though, much experimentation over the years has led to a regimen for perfectly poached eggs.

First of all, use large eggs (small ones will cook too quickly and harden) and make sure they are as fresh as possible (though not laid the same day).

It is also very important to crack the egg into a small container that has a rounded bottom. I find that demitasse cups serve nicely. The egg seems to take on the nice rounded form of the cup and therefore holds together in that shape in the water. These cups also have handles, making them safe to hold while the eggs are slipped into the water as close to the surface as possible. (In a pinch, flat-bottomed demitasse cups, old-fashioned custard cups, or miniature soufflé dishes will do.)

There are hundreds of recipes based on poached eggs. Try them in Brunch Beauty (page 146) or Eggs Florentine (page 18).

Use a nonaluminum pan that is just large enough to hold the number of poached eggs desired. Put 2 inches of water in the pan. (More than that will just give the whites more opportunity to float away from the yolk.) Bring to a boil.

Crack an egg into a cup. When the water is at a full boil, lower the rim of the cup to the surface of the water. Invert the cup in a smooth motion. Repeat with each egg.

Set a timer: 2 minutes will give formed whites and runny yolks; 3 minutes, medium yolks. Beyond that, it's not poached but hard-boiled.

The eggs will start to set as the water returns to a boil. A little of the white will float loosely, but most will form around the yolk. When the water has returned to a boil, lower the heat and simmer for the remaining time.

Remove the eggs with a slotted spoon. Drain on a cloth and use or put in a bowl of warm water until needed. The eggs can be reheated by putting them back very briefly into boiling water.

BASIC OMELET

I like omelets made in the old-fashioned French style, meaning they are soft, luscious, and pale yellow in color. They are not remotely related to the overcooked, leathery, deep yellow and golden brown omelets one is accustomed to seeing in restaurants. My method for making omelets requires some practice, but once you've mastered it you'll wonder how you ever ate the other kind of omelet.

The classic French omelet often has 1 to 2 tablespoons of finely chopped herbs mixed in with the eggs. A more fully cooked or brown omelet can take 2 to 3 tablespoons of a more solid filling. Here is a list of suggestions: Sautéed Zucchini with Dill (page 154), Roasted Cherry Tomatoes with Orange and Cardamom (page 157), Chicken Liver and Mushrooms (page 33), Piselli alla Romana (page 155), and sautéed spinach (see page 18). Remember always to leave an inch border from the edge of the omelet before folding so that none of the filling falls out.

A larger version of this omelet follows.

1 tablespoon safflower oil

3 eggs

Kosher salt

Freshly ground black pepper

Place the oil in an 8-inch nonstick skillet over medium-high heat. Make sure to move the pan around enough so that the oil coats the bottom entirely and reaches about halfway up the sides of the pan.

Using a fork, whisk the eggs together in a bowl just until they are combined well but not frothy. When the oil shimmers, pour the eggs into the pan. Reduce the heat to medium-low. Immediately and gently pull in the lightly cooked edges of the omelet with the fork so that the raw egg flows to the empty spaces and outer edges of the pan. If this does not happen, coax the raw egg to empty spaces using the fork.

When most of the omelet is cooked but there are still spots of raw egg, turn off the heat and flip one half of the omelet over the other with the fork. Slide onto a plate and let it continue cooking for a minute or so. Season with salt and pepper.

SERVES 1 OR 2

VARIATION

For a 6-egg omelet, use 2 tablespoons of oil in a 12-inch skillet. The cooking time is 3 to 4 minutes, and this larger omelet requires a cup of filling because it wants to be fuller and larger.

SERVES 2 OR 3

PANCAKES

Gone are the days when pancakes needed wheat flour, buttermilk, and butter to be delicious. Working from our waffle recipe, these pancakes have none of the taboos but are as good as the traditional ones, and better for you. They are less richly colored than wheat-flour pancakes; but to the good, also somewhat crisper at the edge. The coconut flavor will not be too strong.

¼ cup tapioca flour
½ cup garbanzo bean (chickpea) flour
½ cup potato starch
¾ cup white rice flour
1 tablespoon baking powder
1 teaspoon kosher salt
1 cup coconut milk
2 eggs
½ cup safflower oil

Mix the dry ingredients in a medium bowl. Whisk coconut milk, eggs, and ⅜ cup of the oil together in another bowl, and then whisk them into the flour mixture until well combined.

Pour ½ teaspoon of the remaining oil into a 9-inch skillet over high heat. When the oil shimmers, pour ¼ cup batter into the pan (or use 2 tablespoons to make each silver dollar pancake) and reduce the heat to medium. Cook until the edges are crisp and many bubbles appear on the surface, about 2 minutes. Flip over with a spatula and cook for 1 to 2 minutes more. Transfer the pancake to a plate and put in a slightly warm oven. Add another ½ teaspoon of oil to the pan; repeat until all the batter is used.

MAKES 12 REGULAR OR 24 SILVER DOLLAR PANCAKES

HOT COCOA

With cold winter days comes the desire for hot cocoa, whose powder many of us have on our shelves. The only unusual ingredient here is canned coconut milk, which if you are using this book extensively will also be on the shelf.

The chocolate flavor outweighs that of the coconut, so the taste will be old-fashioned and familiar.

This recipe is easily multiplied.

½ cup coconut milk
3 tablespoons pure cocoa powder
1 tablespoon sugar

Place the coconut milk and ½ cup water in a small saucepan over medium heat. Whisk in the cocoa powder and sugar until dissolved. Heat for 2 to 3 minutes.

MAKES 1 CUP

HORS D'OEUVRE & FIRST COURSES

Into every life a cocktail party or fit of the munchies will fall. They can be particularly difficult as so often the alluring bits of food are placed on pieces of toast, bread, or crackers with wheat. Fortunately, these can be replaced with thin Japanese rice crackers. Word of caution: the crackers crumble easily, which can make clothing a mess if the topping is rather liquid. In such cases, consider endive leaves or other vegetables cut into slices as dippers or bases. Cucumbers sliced across are invaluable. The spicy Chickpea Bonbons (page 181) and Yum Yum Nut Sweets (page 178) can also be great snacks or starters.

Additionally, there are many recipes elsewhere in this book that can be served as first courses: soups and pastas, special vegetables, some salads, some fish and seafood, and other meats. It is mostly a question of portion size. Not all meals require a first course; but they do lend an air of festivity, especially as the table will require more flatware.

It is important that the first course not conflict with or contradict the main course. Balance is critical in ingredients, flavors, colors, and even temperature.

This chapter also contains information on alcohol and includes some recipes for permissible (alcohol-free) drinks.

ZESTY RICE PAPER CHIPS

I love potato chips—British crisps—as much as the next person, but they are not the solution to every drinks party. These, made with commercial rice paper, are lighter and clearly homemade. They last a long time, and the recipe can be multiplied as often as desired and the will to deep-fat-fry holds out.

3 cups safflower oil
2 sheets rice paper
2 teaspoons Lemon Zesty Spice Mix (page 202)

Add the oil to a medium saucepan over high heat. Bring the oil to 325–350°F, then reduce the heat to medium. Fill a large bowl with cold water and soak the rice papers in it. Soak a dishtowel in cold water, wring out, and lay flat on the counter. Gently remove the first piece of rice paper and lay flat on one side of the dishtowel. Fold the dishtowel over it. Remove the remaining piece of rice paper and place it on top of the dishtowel. Blot excess water with a paper towel.

Cut the rice paper into two half-moons, then cut each half lengthwise into ½-inch-wide strips. There will be 30 to 35 strips per sheet of rice paper. The rice paper is quite sticky, so the pieces will not be perfect strips but rather knotty and twisted pieces.

Drop the pieces into the oil 5 to 7 at a time and stir to prevent sticking. Fry for 1 to 2 minutes, until crisp, and transfer to a paper-towel-lined tray. Repeat with the remaining pieces. Season with the lemon spice mix.

MAKES 60 TO 70 STRIPS (3 TO 4 CUPS)

VERY SPICY POPCORN

Come drink time, there is often a need for a spicy snack. This is it, and crunchy too—not for the fainthearted.

3 tablespoons safflower oil
¼ cup popcorn kernels
1½ tablespoons Barbara's Five-Spice Powder (page 202)
Kosher salt
Freshly ground black pepper

Add half of the oil and all of the kernels to a 4-quart pot with a lid over medium heat. Leave the lid slightly ajar to allow some steam to escape. Cook, shaking the pot occasionally, until the popping sounds start to die down, 6 to 8 minutes. Transfer the popcorn to a bowl. Stir the remaining oil and the spice powder into the pot over medium heat until it becomes fragrant, 1 to 2 minutes. Pour the popcorn back into the pot, toss until well and evenly coated. Season to taste with salt and pepper.

MAKES 1½ QUARTS

FENNELED OLIVES

When people stop by, whether expectedly or unexpectedly, in ones and twos or in full-size crowds, I want to serve some food along with a glass of wine or another drink. It is always comforting to have a couple of items on hand that can be prepared easily, preferably ahead of time, and set out on a table with pride. The food should look appealing while satisfying most taste preferences.

One favorite is fenneled olives, which taste better when made a week in advance and kept refrigerated. The flavors combine to give an illusion of sweetness.

> 1 tablespoon plus 1 teaspoon fennel seeds
>
> 4 cloves garlic, smashed and peeled
>
> ¼ cup plus 2 tablespoons orange juice
>
> 2 tablespoons red wine vinegar
>
> 4 cups Kalamata (preferred) or Gaeta olives
>
> 8 strips orange zest, about ½ inch wide and 3½ inches long
>
> 6 strips lemon zest, about ½ inch wide and 3½ inches long
>
> 2 tablespoons honey

Pureé the fennel seeds, garlic, orange juice, and vinegar in a blender or with a mortar and pestle until a liquid paste is formed. This will take 2 or 3 minutes in the blender and twice as long with a pestle.

With a rubber spatula, scrape every bit of the fennel mixture onto the olives. Stir the orange zest, lemon zest, and honey into the olives.

Cover and refrigerate for at least 24 hours, stirring or shaking occasionally. The olives will keep for up to a month.

MAKES 4 CUPS

MARINATED PEPPERS

Roasted peppers are a classic part of an Italian antipasto and can go into pasta sauce or be served as a vegetable. SEE COLOR PLATE 5

> ¼ cup balsamic vinegar
>
> 1½ teaspoons kosher salt
>
> ¼ teaspoon freshly ground black pepper
>
> 1 recipe Roasted Peppers (page 26), cut into 1- to 1½-inch-wide strips
>
> Three 2-ounce cans oil-packed anchovies, rinsed
>
> 6 or 7 chive blossoms (see Note, page 27)

Whisk the vinegar, salt, and pepper together in a small bowl until the salt is dissolved. Add the peppers and their liquid and toss to coat. Let marinate at room temperature for 2 to 4 hours or store in the refrigerator for up to 4 days.

Lay the pepper strips out flat on a large platter. Arrange the anchovy fillets evenly on top. Sprinkle with the petals from the chive flowers.

SERVES 4 AS A FIRST COURSE, 8 AS A SNACK

ROASTED PEPPERS

These have myriad uses: in antipasto, in cooked dishes, and in pasta sauces. If the peppers are young—just out of the garden—they may not need roasting and peeling but can just be stemmed, seeded, heavy inner white strips removed, and cut and sautéed. If possible, choose squarish peppers; they will be easier to roast and peel as below. Diced or cut into strips and stored in olive oil, they will keep in the refrigerator for a week.

6 firm medium red, yellow, orange, or green bell peppers (purple peppers will lose their color when the skin comes off)

MICROWAVE OVEN METHOD

Cut the peppers into quarters and cut out the cores, ribs, and seeds. Remove the peel with a vegetable peeler, being careful not to remove too much of the flesh. Arrange the peeled pepper pieces overlapping in an 11-×-7-inch baking dish. Cover tightly with microwave-safe plastic wrap. Cook on high in a high-wattage oven for 12 minutes or in a low-wattage oven for 18 minutes. Pierce the plastic to release steam. The peppers should be tender but still firm, with a small amount of liquid in the bottom of the dish. Cool to room temperature, tossing occasionally in the liquid.

FIRE-ROASTED METHOD

Leave the peppers whole; rinse them under cold running water and drain well. Roast the peppers directly over the gas burners on medium-high heat, rotating them until all sides are blackened and peeling. Some parts may roast more quickly than others. Check continually and turn the peppers with a pair of long tongs as necessary. As the peppers are blackened, transfer them to a large mixing bowl. Cover with plastic wrap and let stand until cool enough to handle.

Pull out the cores from the pepper and carefully drain the liquid. (The liquid may remain hot for a while after the peppers have cooled.) Gently tear each pepper into sections along the creases. Scrape the seeds and the blackened skin from the peppers. (Avoid rinsing the peppers if possible—a few remaining specks of black won't matter.) Drain the peppers on paper towels.

BROILER METHOD

Heat the broiler with the oven at its highest setting and with the rack on the second level from the top. Broil the peppers until blackened on all sides, turning as necessary with tongs, about 8 minutes. Transfer to a large bowl, cover with plastic wrap, and proceed as for the fire-roasted method.

MAKES 3 CUPS DICED PEPPERS OR 4 CUPS PEPPER STRIPS

SUGGESTIONS FOR CRUDITÉS

With all the peeling and cutting, crudités can be a time-consuming nibbler to serve guests. But they can be made in the morning and kept in cold water in the refrigerator. Limiting the color selection of vegetables to white and green means an easy rather than a fussy arrangement.

2 large bulbs fennel, stalks and tough outer layers trimmed off, cut into ¼-inch-thick wedges around the core so the slices hold together

2 Japanese cucumbers, sliced on the diagonal into ¼-inch-thick pieces

6 large heads Belgian endive, bottom trimmed, and outer leaves removed and discarded, and remaining leaves carefully separated

ROASTED RED PEPPER SPREAD

This quick-to-assemble roasted red pepper spread is a fine accompaniment to crudités. Paper napkins, ice, sodas, and mixers complete the shopping list for a cocktail party.

> **Three 7-ounce jars roasted red peppers, drained, or 5 home-roasted bell peppers (see sidebar, opposite)**
>
> 3 tablespoons olive oil
>
> 3 tablespoons minced flat-leaf parsley leaves
>
> 1½ tablespoons fresh lemon juice
>
> 3 teaspoons drained capers
>
> 2 cloves garlic, smashed, peeled, and crushed into a paste
>
> ½ teaspoon kosher salt

Arrange the drained peppers on a double layer of paper towels; let dry.

Process the remaining ingredients in a food processor or blender until the capers and parsley are very finely chopped.

Add the peppers and pulse until the peppers are coarsely chopped. Do not overprocess. Stop several times to scrape down the sides of the bowl to make sure the mixture is evenly chopped.

Check the seasonings and adjust as necessary.

Serve with crudités.

MAKES 3 CUPS

SCALLOP SEVICHE

I know, I know—it's *ceviche*—but I couldn't resist repeating the *s* to make *scallop seviche*. As written, the recipe results in a beautiful first course. Without the avocado, or with avocado cut into small cubes, it can be spooned into clam shells and served as an hors d'oeuvre.

> **1 pound sea scallops, outer muscle removed, quartered, or bay scallops, left whole**
>
> ⅓ cup fresh lime juice
>
> ½ small red onion (about 4 ounces), chopped medium-fine
>
> ¼ cup finely chopped chives
>
> 1 large bunch cilantro, stemmed and roughly chopped (about ½ cup)
>
> Kosher salt
>
> Freshly ground black pepper
>
> 2 avocados, peeled, pitted, and cut in half
>
> ¼ cup chive blossoms (see Note) if available

Combine the scallops, lime juice, red onion, and chives in a bowl. Let sit for 30 minutes. Add the cilantro 15 minutes before serving. Season to taste with salt and pepper. Divide into four portions and serve alongside half an avocado. Sprinkle with chive blossoms.

SERVES 4 AS A FIRST COURSE
OR MAKES ABOUT 24 HORS D'OEUVRE

NOTE

Chive Blossoms

These pale purple beauties are a rare treat if you are lucky enough to come across them. They are both gorgeous and delicious. Chive blossoms are actually many individual little flowers held together at the top of the stem. To free, grasp the base of the "blossom" with one hand and the purple flowers with the other, twist, and yank off.

HUMMUS

A Middle Eastern specialty that is given depth of flavor by the toasted sesame oil and freshness by the mint. If mint is unavailable, substitute 2 tablespoons of chopped parsley. Serve on lettuce leaves and top, untraditionally, with thinly sliced red onion for color. A clear yellow plate makes a lovely background. As a drink with this, you might try Greek ouzo or Turkish raki on the rocks with a splash of water to turn it milky.

> One 19-ounce can chickpeas, drained, or
> 2½ cups cooked chickpeas (see page 224)
>
> 2 tablespoons fresh lemon juice
>
> 2 cloves garlic, smashed and peeled
>
> 1¼ teaspoons kosher salt
>
> ½ teaspoon toasted sesame oil
>
> ⅓ cup olive oil
>
> 2 teaspoons sesame seeds
>
> 1 tablespoon chopped mint leaves

Rinse the chickpeas, drain thoroughly, and place in a food processor. Process, stopping occasionally to scrape down the sides, until the peas are coarsely mashed. Add the lemon juice, garlic, salt, and sesame oil and continue processing until the mixture is smooth. With the motor running, pour the olive oil into the hummus and process until incorporated. Put the hummus into a bowl and stir in the sesame seeds and mint. Serve as a dip.

MAKES ABOUT 1½ CUPS

BUCKWHEAT TABBOULEH

I love tabbouleh. It is always made with cracked wheat, but I wanted to rescue it for our special diet. This is our own gluten-free version of the popular Middle Eastern dish, made with buckwheat, which isn't wheat at all. When it is a hundred degrees outdoors, this is a delicious first course or even a main with sliced tomatoes and lettuce. When winter comes, I welcome the dish as a side with light foods such as Quinoa-Crusted Chicken (page 87), Basic Roast Chicken (page 86), or Basic Crisp Sautéed Fish Fillet (page 72).

> 1½ cups buckwheat
>
> ¼ cup olive oil
>
> 1 bunch mint, stemmed and chopped
> (about ½ cup)
>
> 3 cloves garlic, smashed, peeled, and minced
> (about 1 tablespoon)
>
> 2 red bell peppers, cored, seeded, deribbed,
> and cut into ¼-inch dice (about 2 cups)
>
> 2 jalapeño peppers, seeded and cut into ⅛-inch dice
> (about ⅓ cup)
>
> 1 bunch scallions, trimmed and cut across
> into ⅛-inch rings (about 1½ cups)
>
> 2 tablespoons fresh lemon juice
> (from about two lemons)
>
> Kosher salt
>
> Freshly ground black pepper

Bring 3 cups water to a boil in a medium saucepan over high heat. Add the buckwheat, reduce the heat to simmer, and cover. Let cook for 8 to 9 minutes, until tender.

Drain and toss the buckwheat with the olive oil to coat. Stir in the remaining ingredients, seasoning with salt and pepper to taste.

SERVES 6 AS A FIRST COURSE, 8 AS A SIDE DISH

GUACAMOLE

This is a guacamole with which I have always had a lot of success, and it has followed me from book to book.

1 tablespoon kosher salt

5 medium cloves garlic, smashed and peeled

3 small jalapeño peppers, seeded and minced (about 1½ tablespoons)

5 tablespoons fresh lime juice

3 large avocados (1½ pounds)

Sprinkle the salt over the garlic cloves and mince very fine, pressing them into the salt with the flat of the knife from time to time until they form a paste. Add the peppers to the garlic paste and mince again, pressing on the pepper, salt, and garlic mixture to make a fine paste that retains all the pepper juices. Scrape into a small bowl, stir in 2 tablespoons of the lime juice, and set aside.

Just before serving, cut the avocados in half lengthwise. Remove the pit and scoop the meat from the skin with a teaspoon. In a bowl, mash the avocados with a fork. Stir in the garlic mixture and the remaining lime juice.

MAKES 2¼ CUPS

SPICY KISSES

These small meringues are very light and addictive. They work equally well as an hors d'oeuvre snack and as an accompaniment to a simple sweet dessert such as fruit or sorbet.

2 egg whites at room temperature

1½ tablespoons agave nectar

1 teaspoon Barbara's Five-Spice Powder (page 202)

Heat the oven to 250ºF with one rack at the top and another rack in the middle. Cover each of two cookie sheets (not air-cushioned) with parchment paper. Fit a pastry bag with a ½-inch-diameter nozzle and set aside.

Place the egg whites in an electric mixer and start to beat slowly. Beat until frothy. Slowly add the agave nectar. Increase the speed to high and beat until the egg whites are very stiff. Fold in the spice mixture.

Now move quickly or the mixture will not stay ideally firm: Spoon the stiff egg whites into the pastry bag. Squeeze out 1¼-inch-round kisses of meringue onto the baking sheets so that they do not touch. Place both baking sheets in the oven and cook for 20 minutes.

Turn off the oven and leave the kisses undisturbed for 2½ hours. Don't peek. They should be crisp and dry. Remove the baking sheets from the oven and slide the meringues, still on their paper, onto a flat surface. Slide a metal spatula or thin ham slicer under the meringues to remove them from the paper.

Eat or store the meringues in an airtight box for up to a month.

MAKES 40 TO 42 KISSES

CRISP DUCK AND FORBIDDEN RICE PACKETS

Duck like the Roast Duck with Forbidden Rice gives very few servings. The compensation is the wonderful stock and what can be done with the little bits of meat that can be picked off the bones. Here is one use of the meat that makes a very good hors d'oeuvre.

½ cup leftover meat from Roast Duck with Forbidden Rice (page 98), minced

½ stalk celery, trimmed, peeled, and minced (¼ cup)

½ small shallot, peeled, trimmed of root end, and minced (1 tablespoon)

½ cup Scallion Duck Rice (page 166)

18 to 20 sheets rice paper

3 cups safflower oil

Mix the duck, celery, shallot, and rice in a small bowl until well combined.

Soak two sheets of rice paper at a time in a broad shallow dish of warm water for 1 to 3 minutes or until thoroughly pliable. Put the sheets one at a time on a damp dishtowel. Cut the rice paper in half and then cut a 2-×-7-inch strip from each of the halves.

Scoop 1 to 2 teaspoons of filling into a tight mound at the end of the strip. Grasping the corner of the paper and firmly securing the filling in place, flip the mound over, creating a triangle. Fold upward to create another triangle, then flip to the right to make another triangle. Keep repeating until the packet is a tightly sealed triangular bundle. Repeat with the remaining ingredients.

Pour the oil into a 3-quart saucepan over high heat. Bring the oil to 350–375°F and then reduce heat to medium. Fry the packets, two at a time, for 2 minutes, turn over, and fry for 1 to 2 minutes more, until crisp. Move to a paper-towel-lined plate. Enjoy immediately.

MAKES 36 TO 40 PACKETS

SMOKED SALMON AND MANGO BITES

Not all cocktail snacks need to be spicy. This mild and fruity one is a case in point. It would also be good at a kids' party.

This delicious combination came about by accident when I was snacking on all sorts of leftovers and random ingredients that didn't quite get used up. We in the test kitchen agreed that, though not expected, this was a delightful duo of flavors. The striking contrast between the pink and gold made it nice to look at as well.

1 large mango (about 1 pound), peeled, pitted, and cut into 2-×-1-×-½-inch chunks

½ pound good sliced smoked salmon, cut into 1-×-3-inch strips

Wrap each slice of mango in a piece of salmon. Secure with a toothpick. Serve.

MAKES 15 TO 20 PIECES

PÂTÉ

Pâté is a classic French first course or in smaller pieces an hors d'oeuvre and is comforting to have on hand for guests or a light home meal. Additionally, these pâtés contain no wheat flour as a binder, which is a common problem as the wheat is unseen. In the Chinese Pork Terrine, the soy is gluten-free soy sauce.

All of these keep well wrapped in the refrigerator for several days (meat pâtés for a week). Whole or in chunks, they can be frozen and allowed to defrost overnight in the refrigerator.

Cornichons and mustard are standard accompaniments to meat pâtés.

PORK-PISTACHIO PÂTÉ

This is very French in flavor but designed for the busy American. There is no need to bother with timers, water baths, and long cooking times as you would when making a traditional pâté—the entire thing cooks in the microwave. This pairs amazingly well with White Bread (page 17) toast points and cornichons. Don't bother peeling the skin off the nuts unless you feel like it. SEE COLOR PLATE 12

> 1½ pounds ground pork
>
> 2 ounces fatback, cut into ½-inch pieces
>
> ¼ pound yellow onions, peeled and cut into quarters
>
> 3 medium cloves garlic, smashed, peeled, and sliced
>
> 2 tablespoons brandy
>
> 2½ teaspoons dried thyme
>
> 1½ teaspoons dried oregano
>
> 1 teaspoon ground fennel seeds
>
> ¾ teaspoon freshly ground black pepper
>
> Kosher salt
>
> 2 ounces shelled pistachio nuts

Place all the ingredients except the salt and pistachio nuts in a food processor and process until smooth. Add salt to taste.

Scrape the mixture into a bowl and stir in the pistachio nuts. Coat a 9-×-5-×-3-inch glass or ceramic loaf pan with nonstick vegetable spray. Scrape the mixture into the pan. Smooth out the surface with a spatula. Cover tightly with plastic wrap. Cook in a microwave oven at full power for 8½ minutes. Prick the plastic to release steam.

Remove from the oven and uncover. When cool, weight the pâté with a foil-wrapped brick (see below). Refrigerate overnight. Unmold. Trim the ends and cut into ⅓-inch slices. Cut each slice into thirds.

MAKES ABOUT 6 DOZEN SERVINGS

WEIGHTING AND CHILLING PÂTÉS

After pâtés are cooked, many will need to be weighted and refrigerated. The procedure is the same for all of them, no matter what they contain. Cut a heavy piece of cardboard—or two pieces if the cardboard is lightweight—to fit inside the top of your pan. Cover the cardboard(s) with a secure layer of aluminum foil. If you can find a brick or knife-honing stone that will fit into your pan, use it. Wrap in foil to keep it from absorbing fat. Alternatively, use at least two filled cans that are heavy and will fit into your pan. Make a place in your refrigerator to store the weighted pâté.

After the pâté has come out of the oven, allow it to cool until you can comfortably pick the pan up with your hands. (Placing the cooked pâté in front of an open window in cool weather helps.) Put the prepared cardboard on top of the pâté, put the weights on top, and carefully place in the refrigerator. Meat pâtés should be allowed to chill for at least a day. In two days, the flavor will have fully developed. If you wish to keep the pâtés for a longer time, unmold them and wrap in plastic wrap and then wrap thoroughly in aluminum foil. Meat pâtés keep for a good week.

CHINESE PORK TERRINE

This delicious terrine cooks quickly and beautifully in minutes. Serve with Chinese hot prepared mustard, hoisin sauce, or even sriracha. Do not make this at the last minute since it needs at least 3 hours to set fully. Plan accordingly and serve the same day to guests, or keep it for yourself and snack on it for a week. The flavors will continue to improve for several days.

  1½ pounds boneless pork loin, cut into 1-inch cubes

  1½ cups loosely packed cilantro leaves

  6 medium cloves garlic, smashed and peeled

  3 tablespoons gluten-free soy sauce

  1½ teaspoons Chinese five-spice powder

  4-ounce can water chestnuts, drained, rinsed, and finely diced

  Freshly ground black pepper

Place the pork, cilantro, and garlic in a food processor and pulse until finely chopped. Add the soy sauce and five-spice powder and process until fully combined.

Scrape the mixture into a bowl and stir in the water chestnuts and pepper to taste. Pack the mixture into a 9-×-5-×-3-inch glass or ceramic loaf pan. Cover tightly with microwave-safe plastic wrap. Cook in the microwave at full power for 7½ minutes. Prick the plastic to release steam.

Remove from the oven and uncover. Allow to stand, loosely covered with a kitchen towel, for 15 minutes. Remove the towel. Cover and weight with a foil-wrapped brick (see page 31). Refrigerate for at least 3 hours, or until chilled. Slice across ¼ inch thick; then cut slices into thirds.

MAKES 108 SERVINGS

VEAL AND HAM PÂTÉ

The colors and flavors of the pale veal and rosy ham create a lovely duo to start any meal. Serving two slices instead of half a slice transforms it from a first course into a good lunch. This would also be a wonderful passed hors d'oeuvre if placed on gluten-free crackers.

  ¼ pound thickly sliced slab bacon

  6 medium cloves garlic, smashed and peeled

  1 cup flat-leaf parsley leaves

  1¾ pounds ground veal

  1 pound 6 ounces slightly fatty ham trimmings, cut into 1-inch chunks

  2 tablespoons kosher salt

  2 tablespoons pink peppercorns

Heat the oven to 400°F with a rack in the center.

Reserve a quarter of the bacon slices and cut the remainder into 1-inch pieces.

Place the garlic and parsley in a food processor and process until finely chopped. Add the chopped bacon, the veal, and the ham. Pulse until coarsely chopped.

Scrape the mixture into a large bowl. Stir in the salt and peppercorns. Cut the reserved bacon slices into 2¾-inch-long strips. If planning to unmold the pâté, place the strips along the bottom of a 12½-×-4¼-×-3-inch pâté mold at 1½-inch intervals. Pack the mixture firmly into the mold. If not unmolding the pâté, place the bacon strips over the top.

Bake uncovered until the internal temperature reaches 160°F, about 35 minutes.

Let stand until cool. Cover with a foil-wrapped brick (see page 31). Refrigerate for at least 8 hours. Unmold if desired. Cut into ⅛-inch slices and then cut each slice in half lengthwise.

MAKES ABOUT 200 HALF-SLICES

CHICKEN LIVER AND MUSHROOMS OVER POLENTA CROSTINI

Of course, classic crostini are made on slices of Italian bread. They can be made on White Bread (page 17) toasts, but I prefer them and find them more Italian on sautéed Firm Polenta. They cannot be picked up, but they can be eaten with pleasure.

¾ cup olive oil

2 batches Firm Polenta (page 171), poured into two loaf pans each coated with 1 tablespoon olive oil, allowed to cool, unmolded, and cut into 2-x-1-x-½-inch rectangles

3 small shallots, minced (about ½ cup)

2 large white mushrooms, trimmed and cut into ¼-inch dice (about ¾ cup)

2 cloves garlic, smashed, peeled, and minced (about 1 tablespoon)

1 pound fresh chicken livers, cleaned (see page 34) (about 1½ cups)

2 teaspoons dried oregano

Kosher salt

Freshly ground black pepper

Heat ¼ cup of the olive oil in a 10-inch sauté pan over high heat. When the oil shimmers, add the polenta pieces to the pan. Fry for 3 minutes per side or until golden brown. Do not overcrowd the pan—work in batches. Move to a paper-towel-lined plate and allow to dry. Repeat with the remaining polenta, adding more olive oil as necessary.

Pour 2 tablespoons of the remaining olive oil into a 10-inch sauté pan over high heat. Once the oil shimmers, reduce the heat to medium and add the shallots. Cook until soft, 2 to 3 minutes, then add the mushrooms and garlic. Sauté until the mushrooms are soft and golden brown, about 3 minutes. Pour 2 more tablespoons of olive oil into the pan and add the chicken livers in an even layer. Cook until barely firm on one side, about 1 minute,

then, using a spatula, turn the livers over and sauté for 1 minute more. Turn off the heat.

Remove the livers from the pan and cut into ½-inch dice. Place the liver cubes back into the pan over low heat. Cook until warmed through, a minute or two. Season with the oregano and salt and pepper to taste.

Put 2 teaspoons of the liver mixture on each piece of fried polenta. Serve immediately or reheat in a 350°F oven until warm.

MAKES 56 CROSTINI; SERVES 10 TO 12

LEMON-ZIPPED CHICKEN LIVER MOUSSE

This smooth and silky hors d'oeuvre is safe for us when served with thin plain or wasabi Japanese rice crackers.

    1 tablespoon safflower oil
    1 medium onion, finely chopped (about ⅓ cup)
    ½ pound chicken livers, cleaned (see below) and chopped
    1 hard-boiled egg
    1 teaspoon Lemon Zesty Spice Mix (page 202)

Pour the oil into a 10-inch sauté pan over medium-high heat. Sauté the onion and liver until cooked, about 5 minutes. Move the contents of the pan to a food processor and add the egg and the spice mixture. Blend until the mixture is smooth and uniform, 3 to 4 minutes. Scrape the mousse into a nice bowl and serve with plain or wasabi rice crackers.

MAKES 1 GENEROUS CUP

- -
CLEANING CHICKEN LIVERS

A yucky job, but it must be done. Chicken livers have two lobes teeming with small blood vessels that are connected by tissue. Spread the livers flat on a work surface and hold one lobe flat with the palm of one hand. Using the other hand, slide a small sharp knife along the connective tissue (at the edge of the lobe) at a slight angle. As the incision is being made, push off the tissues and vessels that extend into the connective tissue being removed. Repeat with the other lobe. Discard the tissue.
- -

DRINKS

I am not an alcoholic; but I do like a good glass of wine or some booze. The wine is no problem for my intolerances; but hard liquor can be, and beer is always taboo. Even when liquor is distilled, there can be traces of gluten, with unfortunate side effects. Drinks made without wheat or barley are generally safe. Attention must be paid. For instance, vodka is usually made from wheat. There are, however, excellent vodkas made from potatoes; choose one of them.

Tequila, rum, grape brandy, Calvados, and the white alcohols such as poire, fraise, and framboise are safe, as are other fruit brandies such as slivovitz.

Nonalcoholic drinks are almost no problem unless they are milk or yogurt based.

Below I offer a very few drinks that are new. I'm sure iced tea and coffee will be no problem. For bottled soda, read labels.

SYRIAN PARSLEY LEMON DRINK

Obviously, in the Muslim world there is no wine with the meal; but the food flavors are strong, and namby-pamby sodas or regular iced tea really don't do the job.

This beautiful, jade-green drink has enough energy to do the job. The ice can be crushed in a food processor.

    1½ cups flat-leaf parsley leaves (about 2 ounces)
    ½ cup fresh lemon juice
    2¾ cups crushed ice
    2 tablespoons sugar

Place the parsley, lemon juice, crushed ice, and sugar in a blender. Purée until the mixture is smooth and a bright pea-green color. Pour into small glasses and serve immediately.

MAKES 1 SCANT QUART

BLUSHING GREYHOUND

Enjoy as a beverage or use as a base for a sorbet.

½ cup ice cubes

½ cup fresh grapefruit juice

2½ teaspoons grenadine syrup

Wrap the ice cubes in a dishtowel and pound with a heavy saucepan. Place the remaining ingredients in a tall glass with the crushed ice. Stir well. Serve immediately.

MAKES 1 SERVING

VARIATION

Blushing Greyhound Sorbet

To make a sorbet, combine 2 cups grapefruit juice, 3½ tablespoons grenadine, and 1 cup Simple Syrup (page 184) and freeze the mixture overnight. Make sure to scrape it periodically with a fork to prevent it from becoming one solid block. Otherwise, pour the mixture into ice cube trays, freeze overnight, and then process in a food processor. Alternatively, use a sorbet maker.

MAKES 1 QUART

RED FLOWER COOL (HIBISCUS)

This drink is commonly enjoyed in the Caribbean, where the dried flowers are called "Jamaica," but I have even had it in the Near East. It is a glorious shade of red. Although the hibiscus is acid on its own, it has a faint hint of flowers that is alluring.

Typically mint is not used but I find that it adds a nice forward flavor to this refreshing summer drink.

Hibiscus with a light honey can also make a soothing winter tea.

1 cup dried hibiscus flowers

¼ cup sugar

1 bunch fresh mint (about 1 ounce), stemmed and chopped (about ½ cup; optional)

Combine the flowers and 6 cups water in a large saucepan over high heat. Boil for 5 minutes. Turn off the heat. Stir in the sugar until it dissolves. Add the mint and let steep for 10 minutes. Strain into a metal bowl and place in the refrigerator. When cool, serve over ice.

MAKES 5 CUPS

PASTA & RISOTTO

These are the Italian gift to good eating. When traditionally made with seafood, they do not use butter. I have included in this chapter other butterless pasta, and risottos to create joy. For information on the rices traditionally used for risotto, see page 230.

While they are called first courses on Italian menus, I find that I tend to eat both pasta and risotto as main courses. Nevertheless, tradition must be honored, and they make wonderful introductions to a meal. Adjust portions accordingly.

Though many of the best wheat-free pastas are Italian (see page 39), many are made in other countries. Look for the noodles—not pastas—that are Asian and traditionally made from rice or mung beans (see page 215).

PASTA WITH ANCHOVY, CAPER, AND GARLIC SAUCE

This is a variation on a Sicilian recipe. It is satisfying without being heavy.

> 4 cups gluten-free dried fusilli, penne, or ziti (about 8 ounces)
>
> 5 or 6 cloves garlic, smashed, peeled, and minced
>
> One 2-ounce tin oil-packed anchovies, drained and chopped into ⅛-inch pieces, oil reserved
>
> 2 tablespoons capers, rinsed well
>
> ⅜ cup olive oil
>
> Freshly ground black pepper

Bring 3 quarts water to a boil in a large saucepan. Add the pasta and cook until tender, 8 to 10 minutes. Drain the pasta. Return it to the pot and add the garlic, anchovies, anchovy oil, capers, and olive oil. Combine well. Season with pepper. Serve immediately.

SERVES 4 TO 6; MAKES ABOUT 6 CUPS

VARIATION

Anchovy Sauce

Increase the amount of olive oil to ¾ cup, chop the capers, and cook with the garlic, anchovies, and olive oil over low heat until the fish begins to dissolve. Serve as a sauce for mashed potatoes, steamed asparagus, or other green vegetables.

COOKING PASTA

All gluten-free pastas will take different amounts of time to cook, depending on the flours used and the sizes and shapes of the noodles. The table on the opposite page summarizes the results of my tests of various pastas from numerous companies, including Schär, De Boles, Ancient Harvest, and Lundberg. If a company is not mentioned, it means the quality proved inconclusive.

I am about to forsake a long-held personal rule and endorse a commercial product by name. I use it. However—sadly—I have no commercial affiliation with the manufacturer. It is a pasta made in northern Italy, developed in the 1930s by a Dr. Schär whose name it bears. This brand can be found online. I suggest that there should be a gold medal struck in Dr. Schär's honor.

This recipe is a general guide. For more detailed notes on cooking times, please see the table.

> ¼ cup kosher salt
>
> 1 pound gluten-free dried pasta

Bring 6 quarts water and the salt to a boil in a large saucepan over high heat. Add the pasta. Stir well. Cook until done to taste or less if to be reheated in a sauce. Drain in a colander. Rinse under cool running water. Add the sauce and reheat.

A Guide to Gluten-Free Pastas

PASTA	AMOUNT	COOKING TIME	YIELD	NOTES
Schär Penne	1 cup	9–10 minutes	2 cups	Looks just like regular pasta, tastes great
Schär Fusilli	1 cup	9–10 minutes	2 cups	Looks just like regular pasta, tastes great
De Boles Rice Penne	1 cup	7–8 minutes	2 cups	Beige, tastes okay
De Boles Rice Spirals	1 cup	7–8 minutes	2 cups	Beige, tastes okay
De Boles Rice Plus Golden Flax Spirals	1 cup	8–9 minutes	2 cups	Beige, tastes gross, does not hold shape well
Ancient Harvest Quinoa Rotelle	1 cup	8–9 minutes	2 cups	Light brown, tastes okay
Ancient Harvest Brown Rice Penne	1 cup	6 minutes	2 cups	Light brown, overcooks easily, tastes okay
De Boles Corn Elbow Pasta	1 cup	6–7 minutes	2 cups	Bright yellow, tastes the best of all
De Boles Multi Grain Penne	1 cup	Not recommended	n.a.	Beige, does not hold shape well
De Boles Rice Plus Golden Flax Angel Hair	2 ounces	5 minutes	1 cup	Tan, tastes okay
De Boles Rice Angel Hair	2 ounces	8–9 minutes	1 cup	Tan, tastes okay
Ancient Harvest Quinoa Spaghetti	2 ounces	9–10 minutes	1 cup	Light brown, tastes okay
Lundberg Organic Brown Rice Pasta	2 ounces	9–10 minutes	1 cup	Light brown, tastes okay
De Boles Multi Grain Spaghetti	2 ounces	Not recommended	n.a.	Does not taste great, does not hold shape
De Boles Corn Spaghetti	2 ounces	8 minutes	1 cup	Yellow, tastes great
De Boles Rice Spaghetti	2 ounces	9 minutes	1 cup	Beige, tastes okay
Schär Spaghetti	2 ounces	11–12 minutes	1 cup	Looks and tastes like regular pasta

NOTES: All pasta was cooked in salted boiling water (¼ cup kosher salt added to 6 quarts water or, for a smaller amount, 2 tablespoons salt added to 3 quarts boiling water).

Schär pasta was the best in general, although the corn elbow macaroni from De Boles was the clear taste winner among all those tested. The De Boles multigrain (amaranth, rice, and quinoa) penne and spaghetti were not recommended as they didn't hold their shape and became quite mushy. The thinner the pasta, the more sauce it required. One cup of ziti or fettuccine used only ¼ cup of sauce. One cup of linguine or macaroni used ⅜ cup of sauce, and 1 cup of spaghettini or capellini used ½ cup of sauce.

Gluten-free pastas tend to be stickier, so must be carefully added to boiling water and must be stirred.

After the pasta is cooked, make sure to rinse in cold water to shock the pasta to prevent overcooking and remove some of the excess starch so the noodles are more manageable and not as sticky.

CHICKEN AND VEGETABLE NOODLE STIR-FRY

This is an ample meal using that Asian classic, rice noodles. Everyone who has eaten it has enjoyed it.

- 1½ ounces dried shiitake mushrooms
- 4 cups chicken stock (any of the homemade stocks, pages 203–4, or sterile-pack)
- 1 whole skinless and boneless chicken breast (about 1 pound), cut in half
- 1 pound green beans, tipped and tailed (about 2 cups)
- ¼ cup shelled green peas (about ¼ pound in the pod)
- 3 tablespoons toasted sesame oil
- 2 bunches scallions, trimmed, white part only cut across into ¼-inch pieces (about ¾ cup)
- 2 bok choy (¼ pound each), trimmed, cut in half between the green and white parts, and then sliced separately into thin strips (keep firmer white pieces and leafy green parts separate)
- 2 teaspoons peeled grated ginger
- ½ cup gluten-free soy sauce, or more to taste
- ½ bunch cilantro, stemmed (about ¼ cup)
- ¼ teaspoon Thai chili paste
- 1 pound rice noodles, cooked (see page 230)
- 2 tablespoons rice vinegar

Put the mushrooms in a bowl, add 2 cups of the chicken stock, and let sit for 30 minutes. Once the mushrooms have rehydrated, drain them, reserving the liquid. Discard the stems and cut into ¼-inch-thick strips—there should be about 1 cup. Set aside.

Pour the remaining 2 cups chicken stock into a 4-quart saucepan and bring to a boil over medium-high heat. Reduce the heat to simmer and poach the chicken for 8 to 10 minutes, depending on the thickness of the meat, until cooked through. Remove the chicken to a plate, allow to cool, and cut across into ¼-inch-thick strips. Blanch the green beans in the boiling stock for 8 minutes or until easily pierced with the tip of a sharp knife. Remove the beans and rinse in cold running water. Drain. Set aside. Add the peas to the boiling stock and cook for 3 to 4 minutes. Remove the peas and rinse in cold running water. Drain. Set aside the peas. Reserve 2 cups of the chicken stock.

Heat the sesame oil in a wok over high heat until it begins to bubble. Pour in the scallions and sauté for 1 minute. Add the whites of the bok choy, cook for 1 minute, then add the leafy greens of the bok choy and the ginger and cook for another minute. Stir in the green beans, chicken, and the reserved mushroom strips and sauté for 1 minute. Pour in the soy sauce, reserved shiitake liquid, cilantro, and peas and cook for 1 minute. Finally, add the chili paste and reserved chicken stock. Drop in the noodles, toss, and combine well. Add the rice vinegar. Taste for seasoning and add more soy sauce if desired.

SERVES 6 TO 8 AS A FIRST COURSE, 4 TO 6 AS A MAIN COURSE

MUSSELS, HEN-OF-THE-WOODS, AND NOODLES

I didn't realize until recently when I found them in farmers' markets that hen-of-the-woods mushrooms could be cultivated. (I have picked them in the woods.) It should have been evident as the Japanese have been growing maitake (same mushroom, Latin *Grifola frondosa*) on sawdust logs for generations. I expect that now that they have begun showing up on restaurant menus they will become readily available.

I have cooked them before, usually sautéing, but they sometimes get stringy, so I decided to try steaming. It worked perfectly. Don't put more water in the steamer as the mushrooms will add liquid. The steaming liquid adds an elegant flavor to the sauce.

> 3 whole hen-of-the-woods mushrooms, trimmed
>
> 1 bunch scallions, trimmed and cut across into ¼-inch pieces
>
> 4 stalks celery, peeled and cut across into ¼-inch pieces
>
> 6 pounds small mussels, cleaned and beards removed
>
> 1 pound rice noodles, cooked (see page 230)

Place the mushrooms in a steamer with 3 cups water (if the mushrooms are too big, cut them in half through the stem end, they will be cut up anyhow). Cover and steam over high heat for 10 minutes. Move the mushrooms to a plate.

Pour off the cooking liquid into a large pot. Add the scallions and celery. Bring to a boil, add the mussels, and cover. Cook the mussels just until they begin to open, about 10 minutes. Meanwhile, cut the mushrooms into florets. Transfer the mussels to a large bowl. Toss the mushrooms and rice noodles in the pan with some of the cooking liquid. Place in a separate bowl. Serve alongside the mussels, and put a bowl for the mussel shells on the table.

SERVES 6 TO 8 AS A FIRST COURSE, 4 AS A MAIN COURSE

VENETIAN RICE WITH PEAS
RISI BISI

This is a classic Venetian springtime dish. It is related to risotto but soupier. I have added a few extra greens for flavor and health. Use enough broth so that the rice is still soupy when served. If cooked in advance, add more hot broth just before serving in soup bowls.

> ½ pound scallions, half the green parts discarded, cut into 2-inch pieces
>
> 2 cups packed spinach leaves
>
> 2 tablespoons packed parsley leaves
>
> 1 cup arborio rice
>
> ¼ cup olive oil
>
> 4 to 5 cups chicken stock (any of the homemade stocks, pages 203–4, or sterile-pack)
>
> 1 pound peas in pods, shelled, or about 1½ cups frozen, thawed
>
> Kosher salt
>
> Freshly ground black pepper

In a food processor, finely chop, but do not purée, the scallions, spinach, and parsley.

In a large pan, sauté the rice in the olive oil over high heat for 2 minutes. Reduce the heat to medium. Add the chicken stock bit by bit, stirring in more as it is absorbed. While still adding the stock, cook for 15 minutes. Stir in the peas and the scallion, spinach, and parsley mixture. Continue to cook, adding the stock little by little, until the peas are tender but the rice is still soupy. Add extra stock as needed to keep soupy. Season with salt and pepper to taste.

MAKES 5 TO 6 CUPS; SERVES 4 AS A FIRST COURSE, 2 OR 3 AS A MAIN COURSE

VEGETARIAN RISOTTO WITH ALMONDS

Actually this goes beyond vegetarian to vegan. I made it for a dinner party with two vegan friends. I used the Vegetable Broth, but commercial is adequate, and the Garlic Broth is excellent if everybody likes garlic—not sharp, but mild from long cooking. This risotto can be stopped about halfway through and then finished. It is ideal in spring, when vegetables are young and tender. I used king oyster mushrooms as they don't get mushy with the longish cooking. Ordinary white mushrooms can be substituted, but they should not be added until the peas are.

I had the idea for the slivered almonds (out of a can) when I was looking for something to add texture and even nutrition.

½ cup olive oil

2 cups arborio rice

⅔ pound yellow onions, cut into ¼-inch dice (about 1½ cups)

¼ pound king oyster mushrooms (see Note) or white mushrooms, trimmed and cut into ¼-inch dice (about 1½ cups)

2 cups white wine

1¼ pounds slim zucchini, trimmed and thinly sliced across (about 4 cups)

6 cups Vegetable Broth (page 206), Garlic Broth (page 207), or sterile-pack stock

4 cups shelled peas (about 3 pounds in the pod)

1 pound asparagus, hard ends of stems snapped off, peeled, tips (about ¾ cup) reserved, stems cut into ½-inch lengths (about 1 cup)

½ cup coarsely chopped dill fronds

2 tablespoons kosher salt, or to taste

Freshly ground black pepper

1 cup slivered almonds

Heat the oil in a 14-inch skillet, braising pan, or large wok over medium heat until shimmering but not smoking. Stir in the rice and cook until opaque or even slightly tan, about 3 minutes. Add the onions and oyster mushrooms, if using (do not add white mushrooms at this time). Cook until the onions are translucent. Stir in a cup of the wine and cook until absorbed. Stir in the zucchini and 2 cups of the stock. Cook until the stock is absorbed. At this point the recipe can wait.

Add 3 cups of the remaining stock and bring to a boil. Stir and turn until the zucchini begins to look glossy. Stir in the peas and the last cup of stock. Add the asparagus stems, the remaining cup of wine, and, if using, the white mushrooms. Cook until the liquid is almost absorbed. Stir in the asparagus tips and dill. Add salt and pepper to taste. Stir in half of the almonds.

Serve topped—the whole or by the portion—with the remaining almonds.

SERVES 8 TO 10 AS A FIRST COURSE

NOTE

King Oyster Mushrooms

King oyster mushrooms (*Pleurotus eryngii*) are long and solid with a small concave cap. They slice neatly and are good for broiling and grilling. They are increasingly available on the Internet and in good stores.

MUSHROOM RISOTTO

The Mushroom Base that's the foundation of this recipe combines white mushrooms with lobster mushrooms (*Pleurotus*) and dried porcini (*Boletus*). Other flavor-packed mushrooms such as chanterelles, shiitakes, or hen-of-the-woods can be substituted—use what is fresh and available. If there are vegetarians in the guest mix, substitute vegetable broth.

¼ cup olive oil

2 cups arborio rice

1 cup white wine

1 cup chicken stock (any of the homemade stocks, pages 203–4, or sterile-pack)

1 recipe Mushroom Base (page 208)

Kosher salt

Freshly ground black pepper

Heat the olive oil in a large pan—I like to use a wok. Add the rice and cook over high heat, stirring, until the rice turns opaque. Pour in the wine and chicken stock. Cook, stirring constantly, until no visible liquid remains. Reduce the heat and add the mushroom base. Continue to cook, stirring frequently, until the rice is done. Add salt and pepper to taste—the amount will depend on the saltiness of the stock.

SERVES 12 OR MORE AS A FIRST COURSE (BUT IT IS RICH), 6 TO 8 AS A MAIN COURSE

SUMMER MILLET RISOTTO

Millet is one of our oldest and smallest grains. While this risotto can be made with rice following the steps on page 42, it has the advantages of offering better nutrition and being reheatable. It also tastes good but is not as creamy as a rice risotto.

3 tablespoons olive oil

1½ ounces (⅓ cup) finely chopped white onion

¾ cup millet

2½ cups Extra-Rich Chicken Stock (page 204) or Fake Chicken Stock (page 204)

2 ounces (about ½ cup) zucchini in ¼-inch dice

2 cloves garlic, smashed, peeled, and finely chopped

¾ cup loosely packed basil leaves, chopped (about 3 tablespoons)

Kosher salt

Freshly ground black pepper

Heat the oil in a 9-inch saucepan over medium-high heat until it shimmers. Add the onion and cook for a minute, or until translucent. Add the millet and 1¾ cups of the chicken stock. Bring to a boil; reduce the heat to medium and cook for 15 minutes. Add the zucchini, garlic, and ½ cup of the remaining stock. Bring to a boil and simmer for about 15 minutes or until the liquid is absorbed. Cooking can be stopped at this point. To complete and serve, add the basil, salt and pepper to taste, and the remaining stock. Bring back to a boil and cook until the stock is absorbed.

MAKES 3 CUPS TO SERVE 4 GENEROUSLY

GLORIOUS SOUP

I'm addicted to soups: hot, cold, elegant, hearty, starters or meals, vegetarian, vegan, and chock-full of chicken, meat, or fish. I have written a book, *Soup: A Way of Life*, about these favorites; however, some of those soups use flour as a thickener, and others are rich with butter, cream, and even have noodles. Others, of course, are perfectly usable.

Fortunately, I have had no problem making new recipes as I cook soup at least once a week and seldom the same one. In the older soups, potato starch or rice flour can be used instead of wheat flour. I roast a chicken (see page 86) at least once a week, and the bones—cooked almost endlessly in water—give me a quart of stock I often freeze to have on hand. I welcome the arrival of good stocks—organic when possible—in paper sterile packs—to keep for times when I'm short. The same pack of tomatoes and a fair supply of leftover wine provide other liquids, as, of course, does water.

I miss homemade egg noodles, but many of the commercially available gluten-free pastas are quite good, as are mung bean noodles, which I often use. I am constantly using my new array of starches. Quinoa is a favorite as it cooks quickly and has a fabulous nutritional profile. All of the soups in this chapter meet my guidelines for good flavor and safety.

COLD SOUPS

These are the delights of warm weather. Sometimes at room temperature, sometimes chilled, and sometimes gelled.

CUCUMBER GREEN BEAN SOUP

This is a delicious cold soup made with seasonal—from my garden—produce. But it uses the veggies that are no longer prime for eating, those passed over while I've had a choice of so many; the green beans that have escaped picking until they are larger than I would like; and the cucumbers that have hidden until they are giants. Of course, it can be made with more ordinary produce; but I like ways of not abandoning my organic productions.

This is a slightly drab green with the crispness of raw cucumber and a hint of spice. It also has the advantage of being gluten- and lactose-free. It can be made vegetarian by using a vegetable stock (see page 206).

Like all cold soups, this should be made ahead to get really chilly. Make as much as possible with the veggies that are available, since the recipe multiplies and divides easily. It keeps well for several days and freezes equally well. Defrost in the refrigerator overnight.

> 3 pounds green beans—no need to tip and tail
>
> 3 pounds Kirby cucumbers, peeled and seeded
>
> ¾ teaspoon Thai green chili paste (see Note)
>
> 3 cups chicken stock (any of the homemade stocks, pages 203–4, or sterile-pack)
>
> 1 cup coconut milk (see Note)
>
> Kosher salt

Put the beans in a large pot and cover with water. Bring to a boil and reduce to a low boil. Cook for at least 2 hours or until limp and soft. Add more water as needed to keep the beans covered. Drain and put through the fine disc of a food mill. There will be about 3 cups.

Grate the raw cucumbers using the next-to-smallest holes of a box grater. There will be about 3 cups.

Dissolve the chili paste in the heated stock.

Combine the vegetables and stock and refrigerate. Stir in the coconut milk and refrigerate until really cold. Stir in salt to taste.

MAKES ABOUT 9 CUPS; SERVES 6

NOTES

Green Chili Paste

I prefer to use green chili paste from Thailand, but another chili paste can be substituted. Increase the amount if you have eaters who love hot.

Coconut Milk

I buy canned coconut milk. A can contains 14 ounces, and many recipes, like this one, won't use all of it. It should keep for months in the refrigerator. Instead of mixing the coconut milk into the soup before chilling it, it can be served in a pitcher alongside, so that people can add their own.

SORREL SOUP SAFELY

Every spring I revel in the clear clean acidity of sorrel. It is available only rarely in shops other than in the spring. That's a shame as I have discovered in my garden, if one is ruthless about deadheading the plants, sorrel can be available almost all summer and again in the fall. A sadness has been that my favorite, cold sorrel soup, has always called for cream. This is a case where coconut milk can be substituted without evoking alien cuisines. The sorrel is strong enough to remain the dominant flavor, not yielding to the coconut. I suggest making at least a double quantity as a dividend for the refrigerator.

Save the egg whites for meringues (pages 29 and 174).

½ pound sorrel, stemmed, cleaned, and cut across into ¼-inch-wide strips

1 tablespoon olive oil

1½ cups chicken stock (any of the homemade stocks, pages 203–4, or sterile-pack), plus more if desired

1 cup coconut milk

4 egg yolks

Kosher salt

Pat the sorrel dry and put it into a stainless-steel pot with the olive oil. Stirring from time to time, cook over medium-low heat for about 15 minutes, until wilted and no longer green.

Add the stock and bring to a simmer. In a small bowl, gently whisk together the coconut milk and the egg yolks. Still whisking, add some of the sorrel and stock mixture to the yolks. Stir back into the remaining sorrel mixture. Heat, stirring particularly in the corners and bottom of the pot, until thickened. Stir in salt to taste, but be careful: salt and acid each make the other taste stronger.

Remove from the heat and stir until cool to the touch. Refrigerate until chilled. If the soup is too thick for your taste, add extra stock.

MAKES 4 CUPS; SERVES 3 OR 4

SORREL SAUCE

Sorrel is a seasonal delight—usually spring. Ruthless pruning and deadheading of the large-leaf French sorrel will keep it going for most of the summer. There should also be a second crop in the fall.

Wild sorrel is a weed in the flower beds, sharper in taste than the domesticated and harder to clean. I used to get my children to weed by promising to make cold sorrel soup.

Use a stainless-steel or enamel pan. Other metals will impart a very ugly color.

Sorrel, a classic sauce for salmon, is equally good with other shellfish and chicken. It can also be used as a soup base.

PRECOOKING AND PRESERVING

3 pounds, stemmed, will give 2¼ pounds of leaves. Cut across into thin strips, it will yield about 28 cups. Heat ¼ cup of olive oil in a large saucepan. Gradually add about 4 cups sorrel at a time. Turn from top to bottom and let melt slightly. Keep adding sorrel until all has been added. Cook and stir over medium heat for 15 minutes or until all the green color is gone and the sorrel is reduced to about 4 cups. Freeze or can in ¼- to ½-cup portions.

GAZPACHO

James Beard wrote *Recipes for the Cuisinart Food Processor* soon after the Cuisinart was introduced into the United States. He asked me to contribute a recipe, which I gladly did. This may be the most often prepared of my recipes in addition to Basic Roast Chicken (page 86). So here it is, once more again, for Jim.

½ medium Bermuda or other sweet white onion, quartered

1½ firm medium cucumbers, peeled and cut into chunks

2 small green bell peppers, cored, seeded, deribbed, and cut into eighths

6 medium to large ripe tomatoes, cored, peeled, and cut into eighths

5 cloves garlic, smashed and peeled

1 cup tomato juice, plus more if desired

½ cup light-flavored olive oil

¾ teaspoon chili powder

1 tablespoon kosher salt, or to taste

Place the onion in a food processor and process until finely chopped, stopping occasionally to scrape down the sides. Scrape into a large bowl.

Repeat with the cucumbers and then the green peppers, adding each to the onion in the bowl.

Process five of the tomatoes until finely chopped but not puréed. Add to the other chopped vegetables.

Put the remaining tomato with the garlic, tomato juice, oil, and chili powder in the food processor and process until a smooth liquid has formed. Combine with the chopped vegetables, cover, and refrigerate until chilled.

Before serving, season with the salt. If the soup is too thick, add more tomato juice.

MAKES 6 CUPS; SERVES 4 TO 6

LEMONGRASS GINGER CONSOMMÉ

This is a jazzier version of a gelled chicken stock.

Sixteen ½-inch cubes peeled ginger (about 5 ounces)

Three 2-inch pieces bulb end of lemongrass (from 3 stalks) and three 2-inch pieces from greener end, cut across into thin strips

3 serrano chilies, cut across into ¼-inch slices

Grated zest of 4 limes

12 cups Extra-Rich Chicken Stock (page 204)

1½ tablespoons kosher salt

3 egg whites, lightly beaten, plus shells from 8 eggs, crushed

1 pound ground chicken

1 large tomato, cut into ¼-inch dice

FOR SERVING

2 tablespoons coarsely chopped cilantro

2 limes, each cut into 3 wedges and seeded

In a tall narrow stockpot, bring the ginger, lemongrass, chilies, lime zest, and stock to a boil. Lower the heat and simmer for 10 minutes. Remove from the heat and cool. Season with the salt.

Mash the egg whites and shells, the ground chicken, and the tomato together. Whisk this into the cooled broth. Slowly bring the mixture to a boil, stirring frequently with a wooden spoon. As the liquid comes to a boil, the solids will rise to the top of the broth. This "raft" will draw the impurities out of the stock and leave a clear broth. When the soup has come to a boil, immediately lower the heat. Poke a hole in the raft and simmer very slowly for 15 minutes. The resulting broth should be crystal clear.

Disturbing the soup as little as possible, ladle it through a coffee filter. Do not press down on the solids. Chill overnight (the soup will keep for 3 to 4 days). Sprinkle each serving with 1 teaspoon chopped cilantro and a lime wedge.

MAKES 7 CUPS; SERVES 6 AS A FIRST COURSE

HOT SOUPS

These are the comforters. They can be elegant or peasanty. All are designed to be eaten hot, rather than just warm.

SPRING PEA SOUP

Simplicity can really be best, especially in spring, when the new vegetables are young and tender. I was all prepared with scallions and mint when I set out to make this soup. They turned out to be unneeded. The soup didn't even need salt, but add some if wanted.

The soup is dependent on tender, sweet young peas and the quantity can be divided or multiplied using the following simple formula. Each 3 pounds of peas in the pod give about 1 pound shelled peas; each pound shelled peas should be brought to a boil in about 1¼ cups chicken stock; after cooking for about 1 hour, this will yield enough soup for 3 to 4 servings. In this recipe, I've doubled the amounts to serve 6 to 8; keep in mind that larger quantities will need to cook longer.

2 pounds peas, shelled

2½ quarts chicken stock (any of the homemade stocks, pages 203–4, or sterile-pack)

Put the peas and chicken stock in a large stockpot and bring to a boil. Lower the heat until the mixture just bubbles lightly. Cook for 1¾ hours or until the peas are just soft.

Pass the soup through a food mill fitted with the fine disc or use a food processor to purée it in batches. Reheat before serving.

SERVES 6 TO 8

SORREL STEM SOUP

I hate throwing food out. For years I pinched the stems off sorrel leaves and chucked them. Then one day as I was cleaning the sorrel, it occurred to me that maybe something could be done with them. I boiled them up, and lo and behold, the liquid in which they boiled had a wonderful flavor of sorrel. At that point I did chuck the stems, but I made a lovely soup—elegant enough for any dinner.

2 large or 3 medium baking potatoes (about 1½ pounds)

1 pound sorrel stems (from 2 pounds sorrel)

7 cups chicken stock (any of the homemade stocks, pages 203–4, or sterile-pack)

Preheat the oven to 500°F with a rack in the middle. Put in the potatoes and bake for 25 to 35 minutes, depending on size. Remove the potatoes from the oven, peel, and cut into ½-inch cubes.

In a large saucepan, bring the sorrel stems and chicken stock to a boil. Reduce to a simmer and cook until the stems are tender and have turned olive green, about 10 minutes. Remove the stems with a strainer and discard; add the potatoes. Bring to a boil, then reduce the heat to a simmer and cook until the potatoes are tender and easily pierced with the tip of a sharp knife, about 5 minutes. Purée the mixture in a blender and serve immediately. If the soup is too thick, add water until it is the desired consistency.

MAKES 6 CUPS; SERVES 4

GREAT GREEN ARTICHOKE SOUP

I had a request to begin dinner with artichokes one weekend. I went to the supermarket; the regular artichokes looked drawn and frazzled. However, there were some wonderful-looking ones with their long stems attached. Of course, they were more expensive; but I got four of them and got even by making a very good soup that was enough for four to six. I added—but it was not essential—2 cups of cooked shelled beans that I had frozen the previous fall. Rinsed canned beans could be substituted. Although healthy, this soup is rich, and small bowls are enough.

> 4 large artichokes with long stems attached, each about 1½ pounds with 10-inch stems
>
> 1 cup chicken stock (any of the homemade stocks, pages 203–4, or sterile-pack), plus more if desired
>
> 2 cups cooked shelled beans (see page 217) or rinsed, canned beans, such as cranberry or white beans (optional)
>
> 1 tablespoon kosher salt, or to taste
>
> 1 teaspoon dill seeds, or 1 tablespoon chopped dill

Cut the stems from the artichokes and cut into ½-inch pieces. With a knife, trim the top 1 inch from each artichoke and trim off the ends and the bottom leaves. With scissors, cut off the tips of the bottom three rows of leaves.

Place the artichokes with stems into a 9-inch sauté pan with water to cover—about 7 cups. Bring to a boil, reduce the heat, and keep at a low boil for 2½ hours or until a knife slips easily into the stems. Add more water as need be to keep the pieces just covered.

Drain the cooked artichokes through a sieve, saving the liquid (about 5 cups). Reserve 1 cup of liquid and save the rest for another use. Remove the artichokes and pass the pieces through a food mill fitted with the fine disc. There will be 3 cups of a thinnish purée. Heat the purée with 1 cup of the cooking liquid and the chicken stock.

Vegetarians could use 2 cups of the cooking liquid instead. Add the beans now if using them.

Season with the salt, adjusting the amount according to the saltiness of the stock and the canned beans. Bring the soup to a boil and add the dill seeds. If the soup seems too thick, add more artichoke stock or chicken stock.

MAKES 8 CUPS; SERVES 6 OR MORE AS A FIRST COURSE

TOMATO DILL SOUP

This incredibly easy soup can be made—except for a large bunch of dill—from ingredients in the cupboard. The only work is stripping off the dill fronds and chopping them. Don't stint on the cooking time or the dill. These are what make the soup special.

I made this for four guests, and they ate it all. So, beware; 12 cups is not as much as it seems.

> 12 cups chicken stock (any of the homemade stocks, pages 203–4, or sterile-pack)
>
> 1 package sterile-pack strained tomatoes (about 26 ounces)
>
> 2 tablespoons fresh lemon juice
>
> 1¼ cups lightly packed finely chopped dill fronds
>
> Kosher salt
>
> Freshly ground black pepper

Place the chicken stock and tomatoes in a medium saucepan and cook, uncovered, over low heat for 45 minutes. The level of liquid will lower by about 1 inch. Right before serving, increase the heat level to medium and add the remaining ingredients. Serve immediately. Any leftovers are good cold.

MAKES ABOUT 12 CUPS; SERVES 6

24-CARROT SOUP

The name applies not only to the base of this soup but also to its vibrant color, silken smoothness, and elegance—enough to open a festive meal. It doesn't get much simpler than this. It is easily multiplied. It needs to be divided to go into a blender. A food processor should take the whole thing.

2 large carrots, peeled and chopped into 1-inch chunks (about 1 pound)

5 to 6 cloves garlic, smashed and peeled

3 cups chicken stock (any of the homemade stocks, pages 203–4, or sterile-pack)

Kosher salt

Freshly ground black pepper

Put the carrots and garlic in a food processor and chop for 1 to 2 minutes. Move the carrot mixture to a 2-quart pot and add the stock. Bring to a boil. Reduce the heat to simmer. Cook until the carrots are tender enough to be smashed with a spoon, about 20 minutes. Pour into a food processor or blender and blend until silky smooth, about 5 minutes. Season with salt and pepper to taste.

MAKES 4 CUPS; SERVES 4

SUMMER VEGETABLE SOUP

While this soup can be made in the winter with canned corn kernels and defrosted small green peas, it is at its glorious best in late summer, when the second round of peas is ripe and the corn is young and tender. The tarragon is a surprising but delightful accent that doesn't overwhelm the delicately sweet vegetable flavors.

If you have extra, it freezes well.

2 tablespoons olive oil

1 small onion, cut into ¼-inch dice (about ¾ cup)

2 large white mushrooms (2 to 3 ounces total), cleaned, stems trimmed, and cut into ¼-inch dice (about ¾ cup)

5 cups chicken stock (any of the homemade stocks, pages 203–4, or sterile-pack)

1½ cups fresh corn kernels, from 1 or 2 ears, or one 15½-ounce can, drained

1½ cups shelled peas (about 1 pound in the pod)

2 large sprigs tarragon, leaves removed and roughly chopped (1 tablespoon)

1 tablespoon kosher salt

Heat the oil in a medium saucepan over high heat. Once the oil shimmers, reduce the heat to low and add the onion. Sauté until the onion is translucent, about 2 minutes. Stir in the mushrooms and cook until soft, 2 minutes more.

Add the stock; bring to a boil. Add the corn and peas and return to a boil. Reduce the heat to simmer and cook until the peas and corn are fully cooked, 5 minutes, or until the peas are cooked through. Season with the tarragon and salt. Serve immediately.

MAKES 5 CUPS; SERVES 4

HEARTY BEAN AND TOMATO SOUP

This simple soup can be the reward for having cooked beans and parsley purée in the refrigerator. I am not being stingy in my serving suggestions: the soup is rich, and more is not needed for a first course. With a salad, it would be a good main course for two or three.

3 cups green rice beans, blanched (about 1¼ cups raw beans, see page 214), or small flageolet beans

4 cups chicken stock (any of the homemade stocks, pages 203–4, or sterile-pack)

Kosher salt

½ bunch flat-leaf parsley (about 2 ounces), washed and dried

2¼ cups tomato purée (homemade, page 208, or sterile-pack)

6 small cloves garlic, smashed and peeled

½ cup loosely packed basil leaves, cut across into ¼-inch strips (about ¼ cup)

Freshly ground black pepper

Combine the beans and stock in a 2-quart pot and boil for 15 minutes over high heat, or until the beans are tender.

Place 2 quarts water and ¼ cup salt in a medium saucepan over high heat. Bring to a boil. Remove the leaves from the parsley. Discard the stems or save for making stock. When the water is boiling, drop all the leaves into the pot. Cook until the leaves are still bright green but very soft, about 4 minutes. Drain the leaves in a colander and rinse with cold running water until cool. Drain well. Place the leaves in a blender and process until smooth (about 3 to 4 minutes), adding water, 1 tablespoon at a time, as necessary to get the mixture moving.

Add the parsley purée, tomato purée, and garlic to the beans. Reduce the heat to low and cook until the garlic is soft, about 7 minutes. Add the basil and cook until the basil is just wilted. Season with salt and pepper.

MAKES 4 CUPS; SERVES 4 TO 6

CANNELLINI AND MUSHROOM SOUP

This is a warm and filling soup for a cold night—even, when accompanied by a salad, as a main course for dinner.

8 thick strips bacon (about 6 ounces), cut across into ¼-inch strips

¼ pound white mushrooms, trimmed and cut into ¼-inch dice (about 1 cup)

2 carrots, peeled and cut into 1-inch chunks (about 1 cup)

4 cloves garlic, smashed, peeled, and finely chopped

2 cups dried cannellini beans, cooked and drained (see page 214) (about 5⅓ cups)

2 tablespoons sage leaves, cut across into ⅛-inch strips

6 cups chicken stock (any of the homemade stocks, pages 203–4, or sterile-pack)

Kosher salt

Freshly ground black pepper

Cook the bacon in a 4-quart stockpot over low heat until crisp. Move it to a paper-towel-lined plate. Add the mushrooms to the stockpot and sauté over medium heat until soft, about 10 minutes.

Chop the carrot chunks coarsely in a food processor (about 30 seconds) and add to the mushrooms. Cook for 3 to 4 minutes, until soft.

Add the garlic, beans, sage, bacon, and chicken stock. Simmer for 35 minutes. Season with salt and pepper to taste.

MAKES ABOUT 6 CUPS; SERVES 4

THE BASIC BEST SOUP

I love preserving the food from my garden and making up new recipes. Even after all these years I have learned a neat new trick. I made a soup with overaged green beans, cooked sorrel, and some chicken stock. It needed some body. In the blender, I puréed the drained and rinsed contents of a can of chickpeas with olive oil and some of the soup. I then combined this with the remaining soup, and it worked perfectly. I am going to try this thickening in other recipes. It is easy and has the benefit of adding a solid boost of protein without any dairy.

Eliminate the chicken stock and this becomes a versatile sauce for pasta, a simple fish, or poached chicken—I call it Basic Best Sauce.

4 pounds large, oldish green beans, not tipped or tailed

1 cup Sorrel Sauce (page 47)

2 cups chicken stock (any of the homemade stocks, pages 203–4, or sterile-pack)

1 tablespoon kosher salt

One 19-ounce can chickpeas (garbanzo beans), drained and rinsed

2 tablespoons olive oil

Place the green beans in a large pot and cover with water. Bring to a boil. Reduce the heat to produce a slow boil. Cook for at least 2 hours or until the beans are very soft, adding water as needed to keep the beans covered. Drain. Pass the beans through the fine disc of a food mill.

Combine the green bean purée, sorrel sauce, chicken stock, and salt in a saucepan. Put 1 cup of this mixture into a blender along with the chickpeas and olive oil. Purée until smooth. Add the purée back to the saucepan and heat.

SERVES 6 AMPLY

BROCCOLI-GINGER SOUP

This is a delicious hot soup for the chill evenings of spring. Don't make it for those who dislike ginger. It has a texture that people think creamy but that comes from the purée and the thickening with potato starch. If you have no potato starch on hand, use cornstarch—good but not quite as.

1 large head broccoli (about 1¼ pounds), stems trimmed of hard bottoms; leaves pulled off; stems separated from heads, peeled, and cut across into ¼-inch-thick slices (about 2 cups); and heads divided into florets about 1 inch at top (about 5 cups)

8 cups chicken stock (any of the homemade stocks, pages 203–4, or sterile-pack)

¼ ounce ginger, peeled and coarsely chopped (about ⅓ cup)

3 tablespoons potato starch

2 tablespoons kosher salt, or to taste

Put the broccoli stems and florets into a pot with the chicken stock. The stock should cover the broccoli. Bring to a boil. Add the ginger and reduce to a simmer hot enough so that there are some bubbles. Cook for 45 minutes or until the stems are easily pierced with a knife. Pass through a food mill using the fine disc, or purée in batches in a food processor—less work, but not quite as good.

Allow to cool slightly. Whisk the potato starch with 1 cup of the soup. Thoroughly whisk the starch mixture into the remaining soup so that there are no lumps. Stir in the salt. Return to a simmer, whisking until thickened. Serve or save and reheat gently.

MAKES 8 CUPS; SERVES 8

ACORN SQUASH SOUP

I have always found it tedious to scrape the fibrous and seedy interiors out of acorn squash before cooking them. Fortunately, I have found the answer: use a melon baller or, even better, a squash corer such as is used for zucchini. This will encourage the making of the traditional squash purée, which can then be the basis for this delightful soup.

This soup isn't too rich to go before a turkey dinner.

1½ pounds acorn squash, split, seeds and fibers scraped or scooped from center

3 cloves garlic, smashed and peeled

½ teaspoon curry powder, preferably Caribbean

1 cup chicken stock (any of the homemade stocks, pages 203–4, or sterile-pack)

Kosher salt

Place the acorn halves side by side, cut side down, in a dish just large enough to hold them. Cover tightly. Microwave for 7 minutes. The flesh should be soft enough to be pierced easily with a knife. Scoop out the squash flesh into a food processor. Add the garlic. Purée thoroughly and for a longish time until smooth. Add the curry powder and chicken stock. Process again. Add salt to taste.

Transfer to a saucepan to warm on the stove. This soup can also be made ahead and reheated.

MAKES 6 CUPS; SERVES 4 AMPLY

DEEP WINTER POTAGE

Come the darkest days of winter, I am happy to welcome a version of that French children's staple, a hearty potage. This one is made with those vegetables that serenely winter over, squash and leeks. I used an acorn squash. The French might ordinarily use a cooking pumpkin.

I change things around a bit by adding some fresh ginger, which gives a warm background taste. I also top the soup with crisp pieces of slab bacon called *lardons*.

1 pound halved, seeded, and peeled acorn squash in 1-inch chunks (about 4 cups)

½ pound trimmed white and palest green parts leeks in 1-inch pieces (about 3 cups)

1 pound baking potato, peeled, quartered lengthwise, and cut across into 1-inch chunks (about 2 cups)

3 fifty-cent-size slices peeled ginger

4 cups chicken stock (any of the homemade stocks, pages 203–4, or sterile-pack)

Kosher salt

Freshly ground black pepper

Slab bacon, cut into ¼-inch strips and fried until crisp (optional)

Place the squash, leeks, potato, ginger, and stock (or water for vegetarians) in a smallish stockpot. Cover and bring to a boil. Reduce the heat to simmer and cook, still covered, until the vegetables are easily pierced with the tip of a sharp knife—about 25 minutes. Remove the ginger. With a skimmer or slotted spoon, put the solids in a food processor and process until puréed. Return the purée to the stock and stir. Season to taste.

To serve, reheat. If using the lardons, float them on top of the soup.

MAKES 7 CUPS; SERVES 4 TO 6

KALE SOUP

A soup that is easy to make, delicious, and loaded with nutrients.

    1½ pounds kale, cleaned, stemmed, and roughly chopped (about 6 cups)

    ⅓ cup olive oil

    9 cups chicken stock (any of the homemade stocks, pages 203–4, or sterile-pack)

    3 Idaho potatoes (about 8 ounces each), peeled and cut into ¼-inch slices

    Kosher salt

Working in batches, place the chopped kale in a food processor and process for 3 to 4 minutes, until almost puréed. Move the kale to a large saucepan, add the oil, and cook over medium heat for 45 minutes, until the greens have become soft and dark.

Put the chicken stock and potatoes into another large saucepan over high heat. Bring to a boil, then reduce to simmer and cook until the potatoes can be pierced easily with the tip of a sharp knife, 10 to 12 minutes. Add the stock and cooked potatoes to the food processor and process until the mixture is smooth and uniform, about 4 minutes.

Combine the cooked kale and potato and stock mixture in a large saucepan and mix well. Season with salt to taste.

MAKES 8 GENEROUS CUPS; SERVES 8

CHARD AND LENTIL SOUP

Most lentil soups are a dull brown. This one from *Soup: A Way of Life* is enlivened in both color and flavor by the additions.

    ¼ cup olive oil

    1 teaspoon sweet paprika

    1 teaspoon ground cumin

    2 medium bunches scallions, trimmed, white part cut across into ¼-inch pieces, plus enough green part to make ½ cup

    1 pound dried brown lentils

    5½ to 6 cups chicken stock (any of the homemade stocks, pages 203–4, or sterile-pack)

    3 small cloves garlic, smashed and peeled

    1⅓ pounds green chard, leaves roughly chopped and stems reserved for another use

    1 medium bunch cilantro, coarsely chopped

    1 tablespoon fresh lemon juice

    Kosher salt

    Freshly ground black pepper

In a medium saucepan, heat the olive oil, paprika, and cumin over low heat, stirring, until the spices are aromatic, 2 to 4 minutes. Stir in the scallion whites. Cook until wilted, about 5 minutes.

Stir in the lentils, stock, and garlic. Bring to a boil. Lower the heat and simmer for 20 to 30 minutes or until the lentils are almost done.

Stir in the scallion greens, chard, cilantro, and lemon juice. Simmer for 5 to 10 minutes, until the chard is cooked through and the lentils are soft. Season with salt and pepper to taste.

MAKES 8 CUPS; SERVES 6

MAIN-COURSE SOUPS

Many soups can serve as an entire meal. The six recipes that follow are meant to.

QUINOA AND CHICKEN SOUP

Quinoa, one of the most nutritious and delicious grains, comes to us from Peru. See page 228 for more about it. With only chicken stock and a little olive oil, this is a soup that can be a meal. It is worth making extra as it improves slightly with a day's wait.

I made this soup after a trip to Syria. It is an authentic nothing; but the combination of spices appealed to me.

8 cups chicken stock (any of the homemade stocks, pages 203–4, or sterile-pack)

¾ cup whole, uncooked quinoa

12 cloves garlic, smashed and peeled

1 pound boiling potatoes, peeled and cut into ½-inch cubes (about 3½ cups)

⅓ pound haricots verts (slim green beans), tipped and tailed

1 tablespoon olive oil

¾ teaspoon anise seeds

¾ teaspoon dried oregano

¾ teaspoon coriander seeds

Kosher salt

Freshly ground black pepper

Bring the stock to a boil in a stockpot. Add the quinoa, garlic, and potatoes and cook for about 12 minutes, until the tip of a knife easily pierces the potato.

Bring 2 to 3 quarts of salted water to a boil. Add the beans. Drain when thoroughly cooked but still bright green, after 4 to 5 minutes. Cut into thirds and toss in the olive oil.

Add the beans, anise seeds, oregano, and coriander seeds to the soup. Season with salt and pepper to taste.

MAKES 8 GENEROUS CUPS; SERVES 4 TO 8

CHINESE GRANDMOTHER CHICKEN SOUP

Well, of course, I do not have a Chinese grandmother, nor would this be her soup if I did. Her chicken would be neatly sliced. I doubt there would be fennel. However, this does make my point that almost all cultures have a chicken soup and that borrowing from one country's cooking for another is endemic. This gradual way of cooking the birds leaves them moist and tender. Serve in large flat soup bowls.

2 small chickens (about 6½ pounds together), innards and wing tips removed and reserved for another use

8 cloves garlic, smashed and peeled

¼ pound ginger, unpeeled, cut into large chunks

9 cups chicken stock (any of the homemade stocks, pages 203–4, or sterile-pack)

1 large fennel bulb, stalks removed, halved, and cut into 1-inch slices (about 3 cups), fronds reserved if desired

¼ pound young carrots, peeled

One 8-ounce package rice sticks or fine gluten-free noodles

Small green beans, tipped and tailed (about 2 cups)

1 large bunch scallions, trimmed and cut across into 1-inch pieces

½ cup gluten-free soy sauce

1 bunch cilantro (optional)

In a large heavy pot, put the chickens side by side breast up, leg end of one next to the breast end of the other. Add the garlic, ginger, stock, and 12 cups water. The water will not cover the birds. Cover the pot and bring to a boil. Reduce the heat by half and cook for 20 minutes. Add the fennel and carrots. Return to a boil, uncovered. Simmer, uncovered, for 1 hour. Let the soup sit for up to 12 hours.

Put the rice sticks or fine noodles in a large bowl of warm water. Stir and let rest for 1 hour.

Before serving, return the soup to a boil and add the green beans, scallions, and soy sauce. Cook until the beans are barely tender. Stir in the drained rice sticks or noodles. Cook for 3 minutes.

Serve accompanied by cilantro leaves and/or chopped fennel fronds on the side.

Serve from a large bowl. The chicken can easily be pulled apart into pieces. Do not serve the ginger.

SERVES 4 TO 6

SPRING FISH SOUP

Well, it could just as easily be called a "stew." It is an extremely pretty, nonfattening main course that can easily be multiplied. Serve with large soupspoons, seafood forks, and a bowl for the shells. Use a pan wider than would seem normal. It helps the seafood—particularly clams—cook evenly.

The pasta is optional. I like to use it at the end to finish the delicious broth. I don't add it to the soup. SEE COLOR PLATE 4

2 cups Extra-Rich Fish Stock (page 205)

½ cup white wine

2 medium stalks celery, peeled and cut on the diagonal into ¼-inch-wide pieces (about 1 cup)

3 medium scallions, trimmed of root end and dark green part and cut across into 1-inch pieces (about ⅔ cup)

12 small clams, littleneck or winkles

5 stalks asparagus, tough end snapped off, peeled, and cut into 1-inch lengths (about ½ cup)

¾ cup shelled new peas (about 3 ounces; 8 ounces in the pod)

12 smallest mussels

8 medium shrimp, peeled and cleaned

6 ounces cod fillet, skinned and cut into 2 pieces

¼ cup tightly packed finely chopped tarragon

2 cups gluten-free penne pasta (optional)

Olive oil

Place the stock, wine, celery, and scallions in a wide 5- to 6-quart braising pot. Bring to a boil over high heat, cover, and cook for 2 minutes. Add the clams and cook until they just begin to open, about 1 minute. Place the asparagus stems (not tips) and peas in the liquid and cook for another 2 minutes. Add the mussels and cook until they just begin to open, about 1 minute. Add the shrimp and cook for 3 minutes. Add the asparagus tips and place the fish on top, cooking until the fish is white on the surface. Sprinkle the tarragon over the soup. Do not add salt and pepper as the amount will vary greatly depending on the level of salt in the seafood. Serve immediately.

Have a bowl of penne pasta cooked in salted water, drained, and tossed in olive oil for those who wish.

SERVES 2

TURKEY CURRY SOUP

There was a weird year when, in the week of Thanksgiving, I cooked a dozen turkeys. My book *Roasting: A Simple Art* had come out, and it seemed that every television show in the surrounding area wanted to see the mad woman roast a turkey in 2 hours at 500°F. The stint culminated with my cooking, nerve-rackingly, a turkey in real time on *Good Morning America*. Then I went home and cooked yet one more turkey for my family.

By that time I was tired of turkey. The redemption came in all the wonderful stock I made with the carcasses—all meat removed—and leftover bones snatched from people's plates. (Don't worry, they boil.) All that has to be done is to cover them generously with water, about 12 cups; bring to a boil partly covered, and simmer for as long as possible—up to 12 hours. I do not add vegetables or seasonings to this or any other stock. I keep it as neutral as possible so that I don't end up with sage in my curry or carrots in my tarragon soup or sauce. Soups made without vegetables are also less likely to sour. That is the turkey stock recipe, and it couldn't be easier.

I never get tired of the wonderful richness of turkey stock, and it can be frozen for later use. This is fortunate because Thanksgiving isn't the only time that I roast a turkey. Each summer I startle the butcher two or three times by requesting a fresh turkey. I find it's the ideal food—not for a meal but to feed late-arriving guests and to have around to be picked on during the weekend: what one friend of my son calls "Barbara's instant leftovers."

The addition of some boiled noodles, peas, and tarragon or some fennel and fennel fronds or some carrots and cooked rice makes good soups. All of which and more started me on my way to *Soup: A Way of Life*.

Recently, I came up with a more unusual way to use turkey stock. I combined it with curry powder. The rich flavors seem to go together very well.

For an even more substantial soup, add additional rice, pasta, or leftover turkey meat. Enhanced this way, this recipe could serve up to 12.

3 tablespoons safflower oil

2 tablespoons curry powder

1 pound onions, cut into ¼-inch cubes (about 3 cups)

¼ pound white mushrooms, cut into ¼-inch cubes (about 2 cups)

8 cups turkey stock

1¾ pounds sweet potatoes, cut into ¼-inch cubes (about 2 cups)

6 ounces broccoli, stems peeled, cut into small pieces (about ½ cup)

¾ pound carrots, cut into ¼-inch cubes (about 2 cups)

10 ounces celery (3 large stalks), cut into ¼-inch cubes (about 1 cup)

1 pound zucchini, peeled and cut into ¼-inch cubes (about 2 cups)

3 cups leftover turkey meat, cut into ¼-inch cubes

2 cups cooked rice or pasta

2 tablespoons kosher salt

3 tablespoons lime juice

Freshly ground black pepper

Add the oil to a 6-quart pot over medium heat. Stir in the curry powder and cook for 1 minute. Stir in the onions and cook for 10 minutes or until softened. Stir in the mushrooms and cook for 5 minutes longer. Add the stock. Bring to a boil and reduce the heat to simmer. Add the sweet potatoes, broccoli, and carrots. Cook for 10 minutes longer. Add the celery and zucchini and cook for 10 minutes. Add the turkey and cook until warm. Add the rice, salt, and lime juice and season with pepper to taste.

SERVES 8

FISH SOUP, CARIBBEAN STYLE

One way to capture the Antilles at home is with a fish soup as good as anything from the south of France, although the Caribbean version boasts the pumpkin-gold color of giraumon squash instead of the tomato-red of the French original. Islanders use rockfish as the base for this soup; I have substituted butterfish, which are much more easily available in New York.

In the Antilles, all fish and seafood, except salt cod, tends to be marinated in the mixture called *bain Antillais* before any kind of cooking, whether stewing, as here, or grilling.

BAIN ANTILLAIS (for 2 to 3 pounds fish and seafood)

Juice of 2 lemons

½ cup dry white wine

½ teaspoon kosher salt

½ fresh hot pepper (jalapeño or Scotch bonnet if really spicy is desired), seeded and minced

2 cloves garlic, smashed, peeled, and minced

SOUP

1½ pounds small whole fish—red snapper, butterfish, etc.—cut into 3-inch chunks, with head and tail

2 pounds small fish fillets, cut into chunks, all bones, heads, and tails saved

2 tablespoons olive oil

¼ pound carrots, peeled and cut into ½-inch dice (about ½ cup)

4 leeks, washed and cut into ½-inch dice

1 pound giraumon (calabaza), peeled and cut into 1-inch dice (about 2 cups)

¼ pound igname (yam), breadfruit, or potatoes, peeled and cut into ½-inch dice (about 1¼ cups)

¼ pound turnips, peeled and cut into ½-inch dice (about 1 cup)

½ pound tomatoes, cut into 1-inch chunks (about ½ cup)

8 scallions, trimmed and cut across into ¼-inch slices

¼ teaspoon crumbled dried thyme

2 cloves garlic, peeled and minced

1 bay leaf

2 small fresh jalapeño peppers, seeded and minced

¼ cup tomato purée (homemade, page 208, or canned crushed tomatoes in purée)

½ cup dry white wine

Kosher salt

Freshly ground black pepper

MARINATE THE FISH: Combine all bain Antillais ingredients in a bowl that will not corrode.

Wash the fish well to remove any traces of blood. Marinate in the bain Antillais for 1 to 2 hours.

MAKE THE SOUP: Heat the oil in a stock pot. Quickly sauté all the fish, bones, and heads except the fillets; reserve them in the marinade until the end of the recipe. Add the carrots, leeks, giraumon, igname, turnips, and tomatoes. Stir to coat with oil. Add 2 cups water and the scallions, thyme, garlic, bay leaf, and jalapeños. Simmer over medium heat until the fish is completely cooked and beginning to shred and the vegetables can be pierced easily with the tip of a knife. Strain the soup through a fine-mesh sieve. Put the vegetables and fish through the fine disc of a food mill. There will be 3 cups of purée and 3 cups of liquid (if not, add water). Add 1 cup of liquid to the purée. Stir the tomato purée and white wine into the purée-liquid mixture. Season to taste with salt and pepper.

Pour the remaining liquid into a small saucepan. Bring quickly to a boil. Remove from the heat and add the reserved fish fillets. Cover and allow to steep for 5 minutes or until just done. Meanwhile, heat the purée-liquid and ladle into six bowls. Divide the fish among the bowls and serve immediately.

SERVES 6

PROVENÇAL FISH SOUP

Some version of fish soup, including this one without any pieces of fish, is made all along the Mediterranean. It is rich and inviting and will vary from area to area.

½ cup olive oil

1 medium onion, cut into ¼-inch dice

8 medium cloves garlic, smashed, peeled, and coarsely chopped

1 teaspoon chili powder

½ teaspoon cayenne pepper

Two 2½-gram packages saffron threads

½ cup dry white wine, preferably Macon or sauvignon blanc

One and a half 28-ounce cans whole tomatoes in purée, strained and lightly crushed

5 cups Extra-Rich Fish Stock (page 205)

¼ teaspoon dried thyme

½ bay leaf

2 teaspoons kosher salt, or to taste

Freshly ground black pepper

½ cup anise liquor, like Pernod

Place the oil in a medium stockpot over low heat, add the onion, and cook, stirring occasionally, for 10 minutes or until translucent. Stir in the garlic and cook for 7 minutes. Stir in the chili powder and cayenne. Cook, stirring, for 1 minute.

Soak the saffron in ¼ cup of the white wine for a few minutes. Stir the saffron wine, tomatoes, fish stock, thyme, and bay leaf into the onion. Bring to a boil, lower the heat, and simmer for 45 minutes.

Remove the bay leaf. Pass the soup through a food mill fitted with the medium disc. Return the soup to the pot. Season with the salt and pepper. The soup can be made ahead up to this point and refrigerated.

In a small saucepan, heat the anise liquor. Carefully set it on fire and allow the alcohol to burn off. Pour the anise liquor into the soup. Stir in the remaining wine, bring to a boil, and serve immediately.

SERVES 5

THE WIDE WORLD OF SALADS

All the world seems to love a salad. I count myself one of its foremost amateurs. Not all of us, however, mean the same thing by "salad." In this country, when we think of salad, the thing that we usually have in mind is a concoction of leafy greens. A little reflection reminds us of potato salad, tomato salad, chicken salad, tuna fish salad, and big main-course salads such as chef's salad and Cobb salad. The world has an even broader frame of reference, including many things that we would consider salsas, dips, and first courses, among which are the Mexican guacamole, Romanian and Middle Eastern baba ghanoush, Asian noodle salads, and French green bean salads. Each region makes salads from readily available ingredients with regional seasonings. I think salads are so popular because they give a solid punch of flavor in a small package and are generally rather inexpensive.

We tend to connect salads with warm or hot weather because they are served at room temperature. There are some salads such as spinach salad made with warm bacon grease that are somewhat hotter, but not really hot.

Actually the lettuce salads are best in the spring, before the lettuce bolts and/or gets tough. There will often be a second good season in the fall. In the heat of summer, it is best to stick to the chicories—endive and the like—watercress, herbs, and other robust greens as well as cucumbers and tomatoes.

With so many salads to choose from, I really had to search my brain for what I think might be some representative ones. There are, of course, no "authentic" recipes as each cook plays his or her own riffs, and even the style may vary from village to village. My recipes come from my experiences in restaurants around the world and from reading many wonderful books about all of the world's cuisines. Also, I like to play and in some cases have taken liberties with tradition to turn what may seem to American eaters more like dips than salads to make them more substantial.

My hope is to give some good recipes and to free the imagination for cooks to create their own salads.

FIRST-COURSE & SIDE SALADS

I remember the days when French friends would come to New York or California and were shocked to have salad served as a first course. Only a few years later, they themselves were serving fancy *salades gastronomiques* as first courses—although they're still not using them as sides.

MIDSUMMER GREEN BEAN SALAD

As simple as it gets, this is a classic.

¼ cup plus 2 tablespoons kosher salt

2 pounds haricots verts (slender green beans), tipped and tailed (about 12½ cups)

1½ pounds ripe tomatoes, thoroughly cored and cut into 1-inch chunks

½ cup thinly and diagonally sliced white part of scallions

½ cup olive oil

Freshly ground black pepper

½ cup coarsely chopped dill fronds

½ lemon (optional)

Bring 3 quarts water plus ¼ cup of the salt to a rolling boil. Stir in the green beans. As soon as the water returns to a boil, boil for 5 minutes. As the beans boil, prepare a very cold ice water bath in a large bowl. Drain the beans and plunge into the ice water.

While the beans are chilling, combine the tomatoes with the remaining 2 tablespoons salt and the scallions. Toss and allow to sit for 20 minutes. Add the olive oil and a substantial amount of pepper.

Drain the beans. Thoroughly toss with the tomato mixture. Allow to sit until ready to serve. Toss in the dill and lemon, if desired.

MAKES 8 CUPS

WATERCRESS, FENNEL, AND ROMAINE SALAD WITH PERNOD DRESSING

This is a fantastic salad for entertaining. It's a more elegant and interesting salad than most people are used to, and there's plenty for when people want seconds.

SALAD

6 bunches watercress (about 12 cups sprigs)

2 large heads romaine lettuce, torn into small pieces (about 8 cups)

3 fennel bulbs, stalks and hard center removed, thinly sliced across (about 6 cups)

DRESSING

1 cup fresh orange juice

1 cup olive oil

¼ cup fresh lemon juice

1 tablespoon plus 1 teaspoon kosher salt

5 tablespoons Pernod

Freshly ground black pepper to taste

Wash the greens well, then dry them. (If preparing ahead, refrigerate in a large plastic bag, undried.) Whisk together the dressing ingredients. Just before serving, place the dry greens in one or two large salad bowls. Divide the dressing evenly between the bowls. Toss well to combine.

MAKES 20 SERVINGS

GREEN PAPAYA SALAD

This is a taste of the French Caribbean islands without ever leaving home. The grated green papaya marinated in a peppery vinaigrette is a wonderful accompaniment to shrimp in the shell or even a whole fish.

Following are Okra with Basil and Hearts of Palm Salad. Some of each of these three salads make a terrific first course.

1 green papaya
2 teaspoons fresh lemon juice
3 tablespoons Basic Vinaigrette (page 195)
12 drops Tabasco sauce, or to taste
Freshly ground black pepper

Peel the papaya and cut in half lengthwise. Scoop out the seeds with a spoon. Using a hand grater or the grating disc of a food processor, grate each half into thin strips and place in a bowl containing the lemon juice. Toss with the juice to prevent discoloring. Add the vinaigrette and season with the Tabasco and black pepper. Let marinate for at least 30 minutes before serving.

MAKES ABOUT 1½ CUPS

OKRA WITH BASIL

A salad that captures the ambiance of the azure French Caribbean waters and showcases the familiar pod as a semi-crisp and brilliantly green vegetable rather than the typical breaded and fried versions that are favored in the American South. Combined with Green Papaya Salad (preceding recipe), it's a good first course, as well as on its own with fish.

½ pound fresh okra, as small as possible
3 tablespoons Basic Vinaigrette (page 195)
1 tablespoon loosely packed basil leaves

Bring 2 quarts of heavily salted water to a boil. Blanch the okra for exactly 5 minutes. Drain and refresh under cold running water for 5 minutes. Drain. Toss the okra, vinaigrette, and basil together. Let marinate for 30 minutes before serving. This salad may be made up to 4 hours ahead of time.

MAKES 1½ CUPS

HEARTS OF PALM SALAD

This salad of shredded hearts of palm mixed with white wine, a little salt, and the green counterpoint of scallion tops makes an elegant meal when served with the meat of marinated grilled lobster.

½ pound trimmed fresh hearts of palm, or 1 can, drained and rinsed
3 tablespoons dry white wine
1 tablespoon thinly sliced scallion greens

Shred the hearts of palm by cutting them lengthwise into very thin strips. Toss with the white wine and scallion greens. Marinate for 30 minutes before serving.

MAKES ABOUT 2 CUPS

QUINOA SERIOUSLY SALAD

My gluten intolerance has introduced me to a new love, the highly nutritious quinoa—same nutrition profile as milk, which is great since I'm also lactose intolerant. It's quick and easy to make now that it is sold prewashed. I cook it and keep it on hand in the refrigerator to add to soups and to go with stews and whatever else I might want.

Today, I was hungry at lunchtime but didn't fancy anything heavy. The ready-made quinoa tossed with just a few fresh ingredients resulted in a vibrant salad that's nutritious, lean, vegan, and delicious. Try it sometime.

> 2 cups cooked quinoa (see page 168)
>
> ¼ pound roasted red peppers with garlic (homemade, page 26, or jarred), cut into ½-inch squares
>
> 1 small tomato (about 3 ounces), cored and cut into chunks
>
> 2 tablespoons olive oil
>
> 2 tablespoons fresh lemon juice
>
> Kosher salt
>
> Freshly ground black pepper
>
> 1 packed tablespoon chopped mint leaves

Mound the quinoa in the center of a plate. Arrange the roasted peppers on top. Surround with tomato. Drizzle the olive oil and lemon juice over the top. Sprinkle with salt and pepper to taste and the mint leaves.

SERVES 2 OR 3 AS LUNCH, 4 AS A FIRST COURSE

CACTUS PEAR AND AVOCADO SALAD

Some of the nicest innovations from my kitchen seem to be the result of happy accident. Once, after finishing recipes for an article on salad I was writing, I was left with a container of prickly pear cactus slices and an avocado. The refrigerator also yielded a green bell pepper. Needing a vegetable to go with dinner, I rounded up these ingredients and made what I found to be a beautiful and successful salad. The bright red of the pear cactus contrasted with the dark green crispness of the pepper strips, and the whole was mellowed and enriched by the avocado.

This dish for two good eaters is not for those with dental problems unless they are willing to spit. The pear cactuses have small seeds like those of blackberries. Eaters beware.

> 1 green bell pepper, cored, seeded, deribbed, and cut into thin strips
>
> Juice of ½ lemon (Meyer is best)
>
> Kosher salt
>
> Freshly ground black pepper
>
> ¼ cup olive oil
>
> ⅓ pound prepared prickly pear cactus (about 12 slices)
>
> 1 ripe avocado, peeled, pitted, and cut into eighths lengthwise and then into ¼-inch chunks

Toss the pepper strips with the lemon juice, salt and pepper to taste, and the olive oil. Add the cactus pear slices and toss briefly. Add the avocado pieces and toss just until mixed.

SERVES 2

MAIN-COURSE SALADS

Come hot summer days or even tired winter ones, a large salad is a happy solution.

CHICKPEA, RED PEPPER, BASIL, AND LEMON SALAD

There cannot be a salad that is more nutritious. I have served it as a first course and as a main on a summer's day.

It is colorful with a variety of textures. Before being added to the lettuce and surrounded by the cucumbers, the salad keeps very well when covered and put in the refrigerator.

> One 19-ounce can chickpeas (garbanzo beans) or dried chickpeas, soaked overnight (see page 224)
>
> 1 red bell pepper (about 6 ounces), seeded, cored, and cut into ½-inch dice (about 1 cup)
>
> 2 radishes (1 ounce each), tipped, tailed, and cut across into thin slices (2 tablespoons)
>
> ½ bunch basil (1 ounce), cut across into ¼-inch strips (¼ cup)
>
> 2 cups cooked quinoa—red is the hardest to find, but nicest in this (see page 168)
>
> 1 teaspoon freshly grated lemon zest
>
> ½ cup Basic Vinaigrette (page 195)
>
> 1 head Bibb lettuce (about 5 ounces), with small, bright green leaves
>
> 1 slim cucumber (4 to 5 ounces), cut across into ⅛-inch slices

Combine the chickpeas, bell pepper, radishes, basil, quinoa, lemon zest, and vinaigrette in a medium bowl until well coated. Lay pieces of lettuce out in a shallow bowl or salad bowl in an even layer. Place the chickpea mixture in the center in a generous pile. Arrange cucumber slices on top of the lettuce in a ring around the chickpea salad.

SERVES 4 AS A MAIN COURSE, 6 AS A FIRST COURSE

SIMPLEST LUNCH

This recipe counts on leftovers and staples, as much of my food does. I was hungry. I had some broccoli left from last night's dinner, to which I added other ingredients, and I arranged them all on the plate in the order of the Italian flag—red, white, green. I put a line of mayonnaise down the center and sprinkled the whole with remnants of my five-spice powder left from a more complex dish.

It was light, simple, and delicious—also healthful.

> ¾ cup cool cooked broccoli tips or other green vegetable such as green beans
>
> 1 hard-boiled egg, peeled and cut into quarters
>
> 1 medium tomato, cut into 6 wedges
>
> 1 tablespoon mayonnaise (homemade, page 190, or store-bought)
>
> 1 teaspoon Barbara's Five-Spice Powder (page 202)

Arrange the vegetables, egg, and tomato wedges separately on a plate. Spoon mayonnaise in a line over the eggs. Sprinkle all with the seasoning powder.

SERVES 1

- -

HARD-BOILED EGGS

> 6 to 12 uncracked eggs

Place the eggs in a 2-quart saucepan—not aluminum or copper. Add enough cold water to cover. Heat to a boil over very high heat. Immediately adjust the heat to maintain a bare simmer (one or two bubbles rising to the surface at a time). Cook for exactly 10 minutes. Drain the eggs and run under cold water until cool. Roll the eggs gently against a hard surface—I cover it with paper towels so it's easy to throw out the shell pieces—to crack the shell lightly without damaging the egg. Return the eggs to a bowl of cool water for 10 to 15 minutes to loosen the shells. The eggs should peel very easily.

- -

ASIAN NOODLE SALAD

This is Asian due to the ingredients, not to my expertise.

> 8 ounces thick rice noodles
>
> 2 tablespoons toasted sesame oil
>
> 2 tablespoons rice wine vinegar
>
> 3 tablespoons gluten-free soy sauce
>
> 2 ounces ginger, peeled, sliced on the diagonal, and cut into fine strips
>
> 1 or 2 cloves garlic, smashed, peeled, and minced
>
> One 4-ounce can bamboo shoots, drained, rinsed, and cut into slivers (about 1 cup)
>
> One 4-ounce can water chestnuts, drained, rinsed, and cut into slivers (about 1 cup)
>
> ¼ pound snow peas, strung and sliced lengthwise and then into thin strips
>
> ½ cup finely chopped cilantro
>
> 1 bunch scallions, trimmed and cut into thin slices on the diagonal

Bring a large pot of water to a boil, stir in the rice noodles, and cook at a low boil for 10 minutes. Drain. There should be about 7 cups. In a large bowl, toss with the oil, vinegar, soy, ginger, and garlic. Allow to sit for at least an hour.

Shortly before serving, stir in the bamboo shoots, water chestnuts, snow peas, cilantro, and scallions. Serve at room temperature or refrigerated.

MAKES 10 CUPS

CURRIED CHICKEN SALAD

This is an excellent lunch or part of a buffet.

> 2½ pounds skinless and boneless chicken breasts, halved
>
> 6 cups chicken stock (any of the homemade stocks, pages 203–4, or sterile-pack)
>
> 2 tablespoons peanut or safflower oil
>
> 2 tablespoons vindaloo curry powder
>
> One 14-ounce can coconut milk (about 1½ cups)
>
> ¼ cup cornstarch
>
> 2 cups walnut pieces
>
> ½ pound seedless green grapes, halved lengthwise (about 1½ cups)
>
> ¼ pound red onions, finely diced (about 1 cup)
>
> Juice of 2 lemons (about ¼ cup)

Put the chicken in a pan that will hold the breast pieces in a single layer. Cover with stock and bring to a boil. Add water if needed to barely cover the chicken. Return to a boil and reduce the heat to simmer. Cook for about 30 minutes, until the chicken is cooked through. Remove the chicken and drain. Reserve the stock and allow the chicken to cool slightly. Place the breast halves on a cutting surface and slice into thirds, parallel to the surface. Cut into ½-inch dice and put in a large bowl.

Warm the oil in a small saucepan. Stir in the curry powder and cook for 2 minutes. Add the coconut milk and a cup of the reserved stock. (Keep the remaining stock for another use.) Bring to a boil, stirring. Turn off the heat.

Stir the cornstarch thoroughly with half of the liquid until smooth. Stir the cornstarch mixture into the liquid remaining in the pan. Cook at a low boil for 5 minutes, stirring constantly. Add to the cut-up chicken, and then add the walnuts, grapes, and onions; combine. Allow to cool. Add the lemon juice. Serve at room temperature or cool.

MAKES ABOUT 11 CUPS

FISH & SEAFOOD

These are some of the healthiest things we eat; besides, they taste good. Ideally, we eat fatty fish from low on the food chain—anchovies and sardines—that are rich in omega-3 fatty acids and least likely to contain large amounts of mercury.

As with local vegetables, local fish tend to be fresher and avoid the use of transport. I prefer fish that have not been farmed. There is some proof that wild fish are less prone to disease. I avoid fish that are endangered species.

It is easy to cook fish if we don't overcook. Almost all methods of cooking from sautéing to baking to microwaving can be used.

BASIC CRISP SAUTÉED FISH FILLET

Nothing is simpler and quicker for dinner than individual fish fillets. The trick is to get them crisp without batter or a flour coating. Rice bran works brilliantly and is very good for the arteries. Think of very simple vegetables with this.

> ¼ cup rice bran
>
> Four ¼-pound skinless mild fish fillets, such as fluke, trout, snapper, or bass
>
> 2 tablespoons safflower oil
>
> 1 lemon, cut into quarters and seeded

Pour the rice bran onto a piece of wax paper, newspaper, or parchment and dredge both sides of each fillet in it. Set aside. Heat 1 tablespoon of the oil in a 9-inch sauté pan over high heat until it shimmers. Reduce the heat to medium and place two fillets in the pan. Cook for a minute or two on each side. Move to a paper-towel-lined plate. Add more oil to the pan and repeat with the remaining fish fillets. Serve with the lemon wedges.

SERVES 4

BASIC POACHED FISH

The Canadians developed a general rule of thumb for cooking fish—whole or filleted—no matter what the method used. It is to measure the fish at the thickest part and allow 10 minutes per inch or a fraction of the time for a fraction of an inch. If time is of the essence, fish can be poached in plain water, but this recipe is for a court bouillon, a flavored poaching liquid.

The number of people served will depend on the variety of fish and the percentage of head and bone. Ask a good fish seller for guidance. SEE COLOR PLATE 8 (HALIBUT)

> 2 cups dry white wine
>
> 1 medium onion, sliced into half-moons
>
> 3 cloves garlic
>
> 5 whole peppercorns
>
> 1 lemon, cut across into ¼-inch slices
>
> 1 carrot, peeled and cut across into ¼-inch slices
>
> 1 bunch parsley
>
> 1 whole fish, measuring 1½ inches at the thickest section

Combine all the ingredients except the fish in a stockpot with 4 cups water. Bring to a boil, then reduce the heat to simmer for 30 minutes. Gently place the fish in the poaching liquid, cover, and cook for 15 minutes (1 inch = 10 minutes; ½ inch = 5 minutes).

BASIC ROASTED FISH

The rule of thumb is still the same: 10 minutes per inch of thickness of the fish.

> **One 4-pound whole fish, scaled, gutted, cleaned (gills removed), 2¼ inches at the thickest point, head and tail on, interior cavity well washed to remove any blood**
>
> **2 tablespoons olive oil**
>
> **2 tablespoons fresh lemon juice**
>
> **2 tablespoons kosher salt**
>
> **Freshly ground white pepper**
>
> **½ to ¾ cup white wine**

With a large kitchen knife, cut three parallel diagonal slashes—lined up with the bones at the body end of the head—into each side of the fish. Cut into the flesh, almost down to the center bone. Place the fish on a diagonal in an 18-×-13-×-2-inch roasting pan. If part of the fish head and/or tail hangs over the corners, that is fine. Rub the oil and lemon juice into both sides of the fish, including the slashes, and into the interior. Sprinkle both sides with the salt and pepper to taste. It will take about 1 hour for the marinating fish to come to room temperature.

About 20 minutes before cooking the fish, heat the oven to 500°F with a rack in the center.

Roast the fish for about 22 minutes. Using two very large spatulas, move the fish to a serving platter.

Put the roasting pan on top of the stove. Add the white wine and bring the contents to a boil while scraping the bottom vigorously with a wooden spoon. Let reduce by half. Season to taste. Serve on the side in a sauceboat.

SERVES 6

FILLETING COOKED FISH

Once you have removed a whole fish from the oven (microwave or conventional), it is easy to fillet for serving.

Gently scrape away all the skin with the edge of a metal spoon or fish knife. This is also an indicator of doneness. If the skin is difficult to remove, the flesh is not fully cooked. Remove the small bones from around the edges of the fish.

Once all the skin has been removed, carefully insert a metal spoon or fish knife into the fish along the backbone, proceed from head to tail, and remove the small bones.

Using two spoons or fish knives, gently push the top fillet off the bones and remove to a platter. Push the bottom fillet off the bones and add to the platter.

Flip the fish over and repeat.

ROASTED SALMON WITH DILL SAUCE

When roasting salmon, as with other fish, allow 10 minutes per inch of thickness. Look at the "Sides" chapter for a green vegetable and, if desired, a cooked starch such as quinoa or rice. Consider adding some extra dill and oil.

SEE COLOR PLATE 1

> **One 4-pound Atlantic salmon, scaled, gutted, and cleaned (gills removed), 2½ inches at the thickest point, head and tail on, interior cavity well washed to remove any blood**
>
> **2 tablespoons olive oil**
>
> **2 tablespoons fresh lemon juice**
>
> **2 tablespoons kosher salt**
>
> **Freshly ground black pepper**
>
> **3 large bunches dill**
>
> **½ to ¾ cup white wine**
>
> **1 tablespoon dill seeds**

With a large kitchen knife, starting just behind the bones around the head, cut three parallel diagonal slashes into each side of the fish, almost down to the center bone. Place the fish on a diagonal in an 18-x-13-x-2-inch roasting pan. If part of the fish head and/or tail hangs over the corners, that is fine. Rub the olive oil and lemon juice into both sides of the fish, including the slashes, and into the interior. Sprinkle both sides with salt and pepper to taste. Cram 2 bunches of dill into the cavity of the fish. Chop the top fronds of the remainder and set aside. It will take about 1 hour for the marinating fish to come to room temperature.

About 20 minutes before cooking the fish, heat the oven to 500°F with a rack in the center.

Roast the fish for 25 minutes (2½ inches = 25 minutes). Using two very large spatulas, move the fish to a serving platter.

Put the roasting pan on top of the stove and add the white wine, chopped dill, and dill seeds. Bring the contents to a boil while scraping the bottom vigorously with a wooden spoon. Let reduce by half. Use this liquid as a sauce.

SERVES 6

WHOLE FISH WITH CELERY ROOT

This aromatic dish looks and tastes as if slathered with cream. It isn't. There is a minimum of fat.

> 1 large or 2 medium celery roots (about 1¾ pounds), peeled and trimmed
>
> ½ cup coconut milk
>
> ½ teaspoon ground cumin
>
> Kosher salt
>
> One 3-pound whole red snapper or other mild fish such as sea bass, cleaned, with head and tail on
>
> Vegetable oil for deep-frying
>
> 1½ cups flat-leaf parsley leaves, washed and dried very well
>
> 2 tablespoons fresh lemon juice

Generously chop off the top and bottom and then the four rounded sides of the celery root to make a cube. Cut the trim pieces into ½-inch chunks (about 6 cups). Cut the cube into 2-×-⅜-×-⅜-inch sticks (there will be about 3 cups).

Place the celery root chunks (not the sticks) in a 4-quart stockpot and cover with water by an inch. Bring to a boil. Simmer for 20 to 25 minutes or until the tip of a knife easily pierces the celery root. Drain. Place in a food processor with the coconut milk and purée until the mixture is completely smooth, 3 to 5 minutes. Season with cumin and salt to taste. Set aside.

Arrange the fish in a 14-×-11-×-2-inch microwave-safe dish. Allow the tips of the head and tail to protrude over the dish if necessary. Cover tightly with microwave-safe plastic wrap, making sure to wrap it under the tail or head. Microwave at full power for 10 minutes. Pierce the plastic with the tip of a sharp knife to release steam before removing from the oven. Unwrap. Use two large spatulas to move the fish carefully to a flat surface.

Skin and fillet the fish (see page 73).

Spread the celery root purée in an even layer on a microwave-safe platter. Put the fish pieces on top in a single layer. Cover with plastic wrap.

Fill a 4-quart saucepan halfway with oil and heat the oil to 325°F. Gently place the celery root sticks into the oil, a handful at a time. Stir to prevent them from sticking. Fry for 2 to 3 minutes, until golden brown and tender. Remove with a wire skimmer, shaking off excess oil into the pot.

Drain the sticks on paper towels. Sprinkle with salt. Set aside.

Reheat the fish and celery root purée in the microwave for 1 minute. Pierce the plastic with the tip of a sharp knife, then remove from the oven. Unwrap.

Standing at a safe distance to avoid splatters, drop the parsley into the oil, a handful at a time. Fry for 5 to 10 seconds. Remove with a wire skimmer, shaking off excess oil into the pot, and drain on a baking sheet lined with paper towels. Sprinkle with salt.

Place the fried celery root sticks around the fish. Drizzle the lemon juice over the fish. Sprinkle the fried parsley generously over the entire dish.

SERVES 4

SORREL SALMON

Here we return to the classic world of French cooking except that the French would lavish it with heavy cream. My husband and I didn't miss it.

As always, use a stainless-steel pan or the sorrel will turn a revolting color. This recipe for two can be doubled, but make sure you have enough sorrel on hand—6 cups of leaves, stemmed, is a very large amount of sorrel.

1½ teaspoons safflower oil

3 cups sorrel leaves, stems removed (save for the soup on page 49 if desired), cut across into ¼-inch strips (about 2 cups tightly packed)

1¾ cups chicken stock (any of the homemade stocks, pages 203–4, or sterile-pack)

2 egg yolks

2 skin-on salmon fillets (about 7 ounces each), cut into 6-×-2-×-1-inch strips

Kosher salt

Freshly ground black pepper

1½ cups cooked long-grain white rice with olive oil and salt

Heat the oil in an 8-inch stainless-steel sauté pan over high heat. When the oil shimmers, reduce the heat to medium. Stir in the sorrel strips. Stir occasionally with a wooden spoon until the leaves turn olive green and become mushy. The leaves reduce down dramatically, becoming about ¼ cup of cooked sorrel after 4 to 5 minutes.

Scrape the contents of the pan into a small saucepan. Mix in ¼ cup of the chicken stock. Set aside. In a small bowl, whisk together the egg yolks with ½ cup of the remaining chicken stock. Set aside.

Place the salmon fillets, skin side down, in a 9-inch sauté pan, making sure they are not touching. Add the remaining cup of chicken stock. Bring the liquid to a boil, reduce to a simmer, cover, and cook for 2 minutes. Turn the fillets over and cook for 2 minutes more, until the surface is opaque. This is for slightly rare salmon; cook longer if desired. Move the fillets to a platter or to plates.

Pour the cooking liquid into the saucepan with the sorrel. Stir well. Heat just until the first bubbles appear on the surface. Carefully whisk ¼ cup of the sorrel mixture into the egg yolk mixture to heat it slightly. Slowly whisk all of the warm egg mixture back into the saucepan with the sorrel. Cook, stirring, over medium heat until slightly thickened, 2 to 3 minutes. Season with salt and pepper to taste. There will be enough sauce for the fish with some for the rice.

Serve with ¾ cup cooked rice per person.

SERVES 2

ASIAN SOLE

This is Asian by virtue of its seasonings, not the origin of the fish. Any sole can be used. The fillet halves are rolled up to make them look attractive and less fragile while cooking than if they were cooked flat.

1½ tablespoons toasted sesame oil

One 1-ounce package dried shiitake mushrooms

Eight 4-ounce fillets of sole

1 to 2 bunches scallions, trimmed, white parts thinly sliced across (about ⅓ cup)

½ ounce ginger, peeled and cut into ¼-inch dice (about 3 tablespoons)

⅓ cup rice wine vinegar

3 tablespoons gluten-free soy sauce

½ cup coarsely chopped cilantro (coriander) leaves

1 teaspoon sugar

1 tablespoon arrowroot powder

Wipe a 9-inch glass pie dish with a small amount of the sesame oil. Heat the oven to 350°F with the rack in the bottom position.

Break the shiitake caps into small pieces into a blender, discarding the stems. Blend until reduced to a fine powder. Lay out a large sheet of paper or aluminum foil on a counter and make a thin, even layer of the shiitake powder.

Pull apart each sole fillet along the center membrane. Pull off the center membrane. One by one, turn each sole fillet in the shiitake powder to coat. Roll each piece to make a paupiette: with the smooth, skin side of the fish out, roll starting with the thicker end of each.

Space the rolls evenly in the pie dish. Strew the scallion and ginger pieces around the paupiettes. Pour on the vinegar and soy and the remaining sesame oil. Sprinkle with the remaining shiitake powder.

Place the pan in the oven for 18 minutes. Remove the pan and turn off the oven. Move the paupiettes to an ovenproof serving dish and return to the oven with the door open.

Pour the contents of the pie dish into a saucepan. Add the cilantro. Bring to a boil and add the sugar. Cook for 2 minutes. Turn off the heat. Dissolve the arrowroot in 1 tablespoon cold water. Whisk the arrowroot slurry into the sauce and stir until it thickens. Remove the dish from the oven. Top with the sauce and serve.

SERVES 6 TO 8

WEST INDIAN CURRY HASH

Without hesitation I stand ready to prepare a hash for brunch or dinner on any wintry day that cries out for it, whether or not the hash relies on last night's meal. And the basic recipes aren't sacrosanct; there's plenty of room for variation. I find this West Indian curried hash appealing because it is a product of two cultures: an Irish dish with a bit of local color from, say, Trinidad.

2 teaspoons black mustard seeds

¼ cup vegetable oil

3 tablespoons curry powder, preferably West Indian style

½ teaspoon ground cumin

1 medium onion, cut into ¼-inch dice

4 medium cloves garlic, smashed, peeled, and minced

2 ounces ginger, peeled and minced

1 teaspoon anise seeds

1 pound floury potatoes, cooked, peeled, cooled, and cut into ½-inch cubes

2 medium stalks celery, peeled and cut into ¼-inch dice

1 medium red bell pepper, cored, seeded, deribbed, and cut into ¼-inch dice

1 medium jalapeño pepper, seeded and minced

1 egg, lightly beaten

⅔ cup coconut milk

1 tablespoon kosher salt

2 tablespoons minced mint leaves

2 cups flaked leftover cooked fish such as salmon, cod, or red snapper or Basic Poached Fish (page 72)

2 tablespoons fresh lime juice

Heat a large nonstick pan over medium heat. Add the mustard seeds and cook, shaking the pan, for 40 seconds, until the seeds start to pop. Add the oil and reduce the heat to medium-low. Stir in the curry powder and cumin. Cook, stirring, for 40 seconds.

Stir in the onion and cook, stirring occasionally, for 5 minutes. Stir in the garlic, ginger, and anise seeds. Cook, stirring, for 5 minutes.

Add the potatoes, raise the heat to medium, and cook, turning occasionally, for 9 minutes or until the potatoes begin to brown. Stir in the celery, red pepper, and jalapeño. Cook, stirring occasionally, for 5 minutes.

Meanwhile, whisk the egg, coconut milk, salt, and mint together. Pour this mixture over the potatoes. Stir in the fish and lime juice. Press the mixture into the pan with the back of a spoon to make a cake. Cook over medium heat for 15 minutes, until the cake is set and the bottom has formed a crust.

Invert onto a large round serving platter so the crusty side is up.

SERVES 6

ARCTIC CHAR AND SAMPHIRE

Most of us haven't heard of samphire, which grows among the rocks along the shores of Brittany and England and looks like a seaweed but isn't. It is crisp and salty. It is also called "glass wort" because the ash when it was burned went into the making of glass. It is a wild plant, although I understand that the clever French are trying to grow it. It is a rarity in our markets. I bought mine online.

Nasturtiums—stems and leaves—or watercress can be substituted, but add salt.

The dish is lovely to look at, tastes just as good, and cooks unbelievably quickly. I served it with roasted new potatoes.

½ pound samphire or other greens

2 teaspoons olive oil

2 fillets (about 1 pound each) from a 3-pound Arctic char (save the head and bones for stock, page 205)

2 tablespoons fresh lemon juice

Heat the oven to 500°F with a rack in the center.

Wash and dry the samphire. Rub the bottom of a 14-×-10-×-2-inch roasting pan with the oil. Make a ring of the samphire from which any black bits have been pinched off around the inside of the edge of the pan. Place the fillets in the center of the ring, the head end of one next to the tail end of the other. Sprinkle with lemon juice.

Cook the dish for about 3 minutes. The fish should be barely cooked.

SERVES 2 TO 4, DEPENDING ON APPETITES

SIMPLE JUMBO SHRIMP

This is a fresh-tasting first course. Or serve with pasta for an elegant dinner.

For this dish the shrimp are butterflied (headless and cleaned of feelers but with shell and tail on) by laying them on their sides and cutting in half—parallel to the cutting surface—from head end to just before the tail.

3 tablespoons toasted sesame oil

2 tablespoons rice wine vinegar

2 teaspoons gluten-free soy sauce

Freshly ground black pepper

24 jumbo shrimp in the shell (about 2¾ pounds), butterflied

24 sprigs cilantro (coriander)

Heat the oven to 500°F with a rack in the center.

Combine the sesame oil, vinegar, soy, and pepper to taste. Rub the shrimp with about half of the oil mixture. Place in an 18-×-13-×-2-inch roasting or broiling pan. Arrange the shrimp so that their shells are up and the fleshy ends are separated from one another. Roast for 2½ minutes. Turn. Top with the remaining oil mixture. Roast for 2½ minutes more.

Serve three shrimp per person, flesh side up with tails meeting in the center of the plate, each topped with a cilantro sprig.

SERVES 8 AS A FIRST COURSE

MEDITERRANEAN SHRIMP KEBABS

These are smashing to look at with the coral of the shrimp and the yellow pepper. They taste good too with the freshness of mint.

The kebabs need to be cooked at the last minute, but all the work can be done ahead. I think rice would be best with this.

> 2 cups olive oil
>
> ¾ cup fresh lemon juice
>
> 1 bunch mint (about 2 ounces), leaves removed and finely chopped
>
> 3 cloves garlic, smashed, peeled, and finely chopped
>
> Pinch cayenne pepper
>
> 16 jumbo shrimp (about 1½ pounds)
>
> 1 yellow onion, quartered and halved through the stem end
>
> 1 large yellow bell pepper, cored, seeded, deribbed, cut lengthwise into 1-inch strips, and strips cut across into thirds
>
> 4 white mushrooms, stemmed and quartered

Place eight bamboo skewers at least 8 inches long in a flat pan. Cover completely with cold water. Set aside.

Combine the oil, lemon juice, mint, garlic, and cayenne and mix well to make a marinade. Add the remaining ingredients and marinate for 30 minutes.

Heat the broiler with the rack at the top. To assemble the kebabs, slide a skewer through a mushroom quarter, pepper piece, shrimp, onion piece, shrimp, pepper, and mushroom again. Repeat with the remaining seven skewers.

Rub 1½ tablespoons of the marinade on the bottom of a shallow 16-×-11-inch roasting pan. Put in the skewers in an even layer. Broil for 2 minutes, then turn the skewers over and broil for 3 minutes more. Serve immediately.

SERVES 8 AS A FIRST COURSE, 4 AS A MAIN COURSE

SALMON SHIITAKE KEBABS

These are the kebabs for which I developed the Green Velvet Cilantro Sauce, and I have served them as a first and a main course. Continuing the theme of not discarding, I used sticks cut lengthwise from the hard core of a pineapple as the skewers. Of course, regular skewers will work just as well.

> 1½ pounds skinless and boneless salmon, cut into 1-inch cubes (about 30)
>
> ½ pound (8 whole) fresh shiitake mushrooms, stems removed and caps cut into quarters, or, if using dried, soaked in hot water for 30 minutes
>
> ½ recipe Green Velvet Cilantro Sauce (page 194)
>
> 1½ tablespoons safflower oil

Prepare eight pineapple skewers according to the directions on page 185. If using bamboo skewers, place them in a flat pan and cover with cold water for at least 1 hour before using.

Pierce the salmon cubes and shiitake quarters, alternating between the two. Each skewer should have three or four pieces of salmon and four pieces of mushroom. Place them in the bottom of a large roasting pan or casserole dish. Coat each skewer with the sauce. Cover with plastic wrap and refrigerate for 30 minutes, turning the skewers over halfway through. Heat the broiler and place a rack at the top of the oven.

Coat the bottom of a separate large roasting pan with the safflower oil. Put the skewers in the pan, spacing them evenly so they do not touch. Pour the marinade from the original pan over the skewers and broil for 2 to 3 minutes per side.

SERVES 8 AS A FIRST COURSE, 4 AS A MAIN COURSE

MARINATED SHRIMP, MUSSELS, AND ARTICHOKE HEARTS

This sprightly marinated seafood can be prepared the day before, making it an ideal starter for a party.

Four 9-ounce boxes frozen artichoke hearts

6½ pounds mussels (about 6 dozen), scrubbed and beards removed

1 teaspoon kosher salt

3¼ pounds medium shrimp (20 to 24 to the pound), shelled

8 stalks celery (about 1½ pounds), peeled and cut diagonally into ¼-inch slices

¾ pound white onions, quartered and thinly sliced (2 cups)

MARINADE

½ cup fresh lemon juice

¼ cup good-quality olive oil

1 tablespoon kosher salt

½ teaspoon freshly ground black pepper

¼ cup drained and rinsed capers

¾ cup liquid from cooked mussels

Open the boxes of artichoke hearts. Place the artichokes in a sieve under hot running water until they can be separated. Place in a bowl of hot water until thoroughly defrosted. Drain. Set aside.

Put the mussels with ¼ cup water in a large pot with a tight-fitting lid. Cook for 10 minutes, shaking the pot—holding the cover on—once during the cooking. Remove from the heat. Allow to cool until the mussels can be handled. Shell the mussels, using one shell as tweezers. Place the meat in a very large bowl. Discard the shells. Strain the mussel liquid through a sieve lined with a damp cloth. Reserve.

Bring 3 quarts water with the salt to a boil in a large pot. Drop in the shrimp. Stir. Cover the pot and turn off the heat. Let the shrimp steep for 5 minutes. Drain in a large colander. In a large bowl, combine the shrimp, mussels, artichokes, celery, and onions.

Whisk together the marinade ingredients. Pour over the salad. With hands or large spoons, mix thoroughly. Cover the bowl with plastic wrap and refrigerate. Stir once or twice before dinner.

MAKES 20 SERVINGS AS A FIRST COURSE, 10 AS A MAIN COURSE

POMEGRANATE SHRIMP SAUTÉ WITH FRISÉE

Pomegranate juice is now readily available in groceries. But it is almost just as easy to buy some large dark red heavy pomegranates and juice them yourself, extracting the beautiful seeds, to make similar dishes or new ones.

The flavor of pomegranate and the beauty of its seeds go well in any part of a meal. The shrimp dish here, a lovely first course, uses plenty of spice but is not, as one might think, hot. The pomegranate provides color, crispness, and fresh flavor.

2 tablespoons toasted sesame oil

2 tablespoons vegetable oil

2 tablespoons coriander seeds

2 tablespoons ground cumin

Freshly ground black pepper

1 tablespoon black mustard seeds

2 medium shallots, minced

30 large shrimp (1¼ pounds), peeled and deveined

Juice from 1 large or 2 small ripe pomegranates (½ cup; see sidebar, right)

1 tablespoon red wine vinegar

1 teaspoon kosher salt

½ pound light-colored frisée (chicory), heavy stems removed, leaf portion torn into 2-inch pieces (2 packed cups)

Seeds from ¼ large or ½ small pomegranate (about 2 tablespoons; see sidebar, right)

In a 12-inch skillet, combine a tablespoon of the sesame oil with the vegetable oil, coriander seeds, cumin, pepper to taste, and black mustard seeds. Place over medium heat and cook, stirring, for 3 minutes. Stir in the shallots and cook, stirring, for 4 minutes.

Raise the heat to high. Stir in the shrimp, and cook, turning and stirring, for 3 minutes, or until the shrimp are opaque.

Reduce the heat to medium-low. Stir in the pomegranate juice, vinegar, and salt. Cook, stirring and scraping the bottom of the pan, for 1 minute. Stir in the remaining sesame oil.

Place ½ cup frisée on each plate. Top with shrimp and drizzle the sauce around the plate. Sprinkle with pomegranate seeds.

SERVES 4 AS A FIRST COURSE

USING FRESH POMEGRANATES

TO JUICE A POMEGRANATE

First cut it in half horizontally between the stem and blossom end. Holding one half over a bowl, use a citrus juicer—an electric one is easier—to extract the maximum amount of juice. A large ripe pomegranate will produce ½ cup of juice; a small one will give as little as ¼ cup.

TO SEED A POMEGRANATE

Cut it into quarters. Working over a bowl, use a small spoon or your fingers to gently pull the seeds away from the pulp. (The juice may stain your fingers temporarily, but it washes off easily.) The seeds are fragile, so take care to keep them whole. As the seeds are pulled away, they separate from each other. Drop the seeds into a measuring cup and pick off any white membrane clinging to them. A large pomegranate will yield 1 cup to 1½ cups seeds; a small one will yield ½ to ¾ cup. (If you end up with more seeds than you need for a recipe, sprinkle them over a fruit or green salad for color and crispness.)

SEA SCALLOPS WITH SALMON CAVIAR SAUCE

This is a very pretty, festive dish that was approved by two of my fussiest gourmet friends. It needn't be poisonously expensive if the salmon caviar is bought jarred. Do look at the general instructions for mayonnaise on page 190.

12 large sea scallops with side muscle removed and reserved

½ teaspoon plus 1 cup olive oil

½ cup (one 4-ounce jar) salmon roe

¼ cup fresh lemon juice

Put the reserved muscle pieces into the water that will go under a steamer tray. Grease the upper surface of the steamer tray with the ½ teaspoon oil. Lay the scallops on the steamer in a single layer. Bring the water to a boil without the steamer tray.

Put the roe in a blender with the lemon juice. Blend until smooth. Remove the cap—not the top—from the blender. Pour in the remaining olive oil in a steady stream with the motor running. Place the desired amount of sauce in the center of a plate for each person. I used about ⅓ cup per person.

Just before serving, place the steamer tray over the water and cover the steamer. Cook the scallops just until white or opaque, about 3 minutes. Place three scallops around each blob of sauce. Serve with a sauce spoon if available.

Any extra sauce can be refrigerated for up to 3 days and can be served with any simple fish.

SERVES 4 AS A FIRST COURSE

CHICKEN & OTHER BIRDS

Chicken may be the world's favorite animal protein. Certainly, it is one of mine. Low in calories, they are healthy and free range chickens (no chemicals) are certainly better.

During World War II, my contribution—unwilling—to the war effort was taking care of a brood of chickens: feeding them, mucking out the hen house, and retrieving the eggs. It didn't seem to make them any friendlier that I was feeding them twice a day. I also learned how realistic the term "pecking order" is. The flock will select one bird and literally peck it to death if they are not stopped, which means isolating the benighted animal.

I have seen photographs in the popular press of some small child cuddling a pet chicken. I never could understand it.

In addition to my signature roast chickens, there are some delicious recipes in the following pages, especially those for stews, which traditionally require flour, butter, and cream—but, as I discovered, really do not.

Besides chicken, myriad other birds are delicious. I cover a few of them here, but this section is hardly exhaustive, especially when it comes to game birds. The ardent cook might want to take a look at my book *Roasting: A Simple Art* for other possibilities.

BASIC ROAST CHICKEN

One of my versions of this recipe is the most popular thing that I have ever written, closely followed by Basic Roast Turkey (page 95). Along with variations, it is in my other books, but I include it again here because this book would be incomplete without it.

I make one almost every week, and the carcass and innards—not the liver—provide the makings of the often-needed chicken stock (pages 203–4).

This is family fare and company fare. The chickens can range in size from about 3½ pounds to 6 pounds. I often make two smaller chickens in the same pan, neck end abutting butt end. It's not so much that the smaller birds roast more quickly but that two birds gives a better shot at each person's getting his or her favorite piece of the bird.

In any case, the chicken will take about 10 minutes a pound by my method. Two at a time will take no more than one, but enough space should be allowed in the pan so that they do not touch.

I like tarragon in the deglazing sauce or, for a more emphatic touch, a little harissa.

One 5- to 6-pound chicken at room temperature, wing tips removed

1 lemon, halved

4 whole garlic cloves

Kosher salt

Freshly ground black pepper

1 cup chicken stock (any of the homemade stocks, pages 203–4, or sterile-pack)

Heat the oven to 500°F with a rack on the second level from the bottom. Remove the fat from the tail and crop end of the chicken. Freeze the neck and giblets for chicken stock. Reserve the chicken livers for another use, such as pâté (see pages 33 and 34).

Put the chicken in a roasting pan no more than 2½ inches deep. Choose a pan that just holds the chicken or has room for potatoes or other vegetables that may well surround it. Squeeze the lemon juice over the chicken. Stuff the cavity of the chicken with the lemon shells and garlic. Season the cavity with salt and pepper to taste. Place the chicken in the roasting pan breast side up.

Put in the oven legs first and roast for 50 to 60 minutes, or until the juices run clear. After the first 10 minutes, move the chicken with a wooden spoon to prevent it from sticking.

Move the chicken to a platter by placing a large wooden spoon into the tail end and balancing the chicken with a kitchen spoon pressed against the neck end. As you lift the chicken, tilt it over the roasting pan so that all the juices run out into the pan.

Pour off or spoon out excess fat from the roasting pan and put the roasting pan on top of the stove. Add the stock and bring the contents of the pan to a boil while scraping the bottom vigorously with a wooden spoon. Let reduce by half. Serve the sauce over the chicken or, for crisp skin, in a sauceboat.

SERVES 4 TO 6 AS A MAIN COURSE

ROAST CHICKEN WITH GARLIC SAUCE

I love garlic when it has cooked long enough to lose some of its raw taste and even more when with longer cooking it turns sweet. The two methods of cooking make perfection.

> One 5-pound chicken at room temperature, wing tips removed
>
> 3 heads garlic, smashed, cloves separated, and peeled
>
> 1¼ cups chicken stock (any of the homemade stocks, pages 203–4, or sterile-pack)
>
> 1¼ teaspoons kosher salt
>
> 1 tablespoon plus 1 teaspoon fresh lemon juice

Heat the oven to 500°F, with a rack on the second level from the bottom. Remove the fat from the tail and crop end of the chicken. Freeze the neck and giblets for chicken stock. Reserve the chicken livers for another use, such as pâté (pages 33 and 34).

Place the chicken in a 12-×-8-×-1½-inch roasting pan breast side up. Put in the oven legs first and roast for 50 to 60 minutes or until the juices run clear. After the first 10 minutes, move the chicken with a wooden spoon to keep it from sticking. Twenty minutes before the chicken is done, add the garlic to the pan, making sure to stir the cloves around in the rendered fat.

At the end of the cooking time, move the chicken to a platter by placing a large wooden spoon into the tail end and balancing the chicken with a kitchen spoon pressed against the neck. Tilt the chicken over the roasting pan as it is being transferred so that all the juices run into it.

Put the roasting pan on the stove. Add ½ cup stock and bring to a boil while scraping the bottom vigorously with a wooden spoon. Scrape all the contents of the pan into a food processor. Add the remaining stock. Blend until smooth, about 3 minutes. Season with the salt and lemon juice. Serve immediately with the chicken.

SERVES 4; MAKES SCANT 2 CUPS GARLIC SAUCE

QUINOA-CRUSTED CHICKEN

Almost all of us have eaten chicken lightly coated with flour before sautéing. The flour keeps the chicken moist and gives it a nice light crust. The perfect solution to the flour problem is quinoa. For this use I prefer the fancy almost-white quinoa.

> ½ cup chicken stock (any of the homemade stocks, pages 203–4, or sterile-pack)
>
> 1 cup whole, uncooked quinoa
>
> 2 skinless and boneless chicken breasts (about 2 pounds)
>
> ¼ cup plus 2 tablespoons vegetable oil
>
> Kosher salt
>
> Freshly ground black pepper
>
> ½ lemon, cut lengthwise into 8 wedges

Pour the chicken stock into a wide bowl. Place the quinoa on a large flat dinner plate. Set both aside.

Place a chicken breast flat on a cutting board skinned side up. Cut in half down the middle. Turn each half over and pull off the strip of flesh that is the chicken tender. Wrap the tenders in plastic wrap or foil. Set aside. Repeat with the other breast piece.

One half-breast at a time, put your palm flat on each piece. Slide a knife parallel to the cutting board through the chicken, resulting in two thin cutlets from each half-breast. There will be eight cutlets total.

Heat 1½ tablespoons of the oil in a large pan over high heat until slightly blue but not smoking. In the meantime, dip both sides of two pieces of breast into the stock. Then, one at a time, dip both sides of the breast pieces into the quinoa. Reduce the oil heat to medium and place a pair of chicken pieces next to each other in the hot oil. Cook for 2 to 3 minutes per side, until the flesh turns opaque. Move the cooked pieces to plates or a platter. Season with salt and pepper to taste. Repeat with the remaining chicken pieces. Serve with the lemon wedges.

SERVES 4

CHINESE CHICKEN IN THE POT

The comfortable standby chicken in the pot varies with readily available Chinese ingredients, like star anise and ginger. They perfume the soup, lift the taste, and compensate for the lack of deep flavor if using canned broth. Buying chicken cut into pieces makes the cooking go more quickly. Having it on the bone gives the soup more flavor and body. And skinning it not only drastically reduces the fat but also eliminates the waxen dead-looking cooked skin in each portion. Many butchers and supermarkets will skin the chicken. If not, it is easily removed by slipping a finger or two under the skin of each piece and pulling it off.

Rather than putting the rice into the soup, it can be put into a heavy earthenware container with a lid. This keeps it warm and lets guests add their own, usually after they have cut the chicken from the bone. The next day, the chicken can be cut into strips from the bone and stirred into the soup along with the rice for a first course.

> 8 cups chicken stock (any of the homemade stocks, pages 203–4, or sterile-pack)
>
> 1 ounce dried shiitake mushrooms
>
> Two 4-pound chickens, each cut into 8 serving pieces and skinned, excess visible fat removed and backs, necks, and wing tips reserved for another use
>
> 8 cloves garlic, smashed and peeled
>
> 1½ inches ginger, peeled and cut across into ⅛-inch-thick slices and then into thin strips
>
> 2 whole star anise or 1 heaping tablespoon star anise pieces
>
> ½ cup gluten-free soy sauce
>
> 2 bunches scallions, trimmed, white part cut into 2-inch lengths, and half of the greens cut into 2-inch lengths (1 cup greens)
>
> Two 8-ounce cans sliced water chestnuts, drained and rinsed well under cold water
>
> 6 ounces snow peas, tipped and tailed
>
> 6 cups cooked white rice

Heat 2 cups of the stock until warm, soak the mushrooms in the warm stock for 15 minutes, and drain; strain the liquid through a coffee filter and reserve.

Place the chicken, the remaining 6 cups stock, the garlic, ginger, and star anise in a large wide pot. Cover. Bring to a boil.

Add the mushroom liquid and soy sauce. When the liquid returns to a moderate boil, add the scallion whites and mushrooms. Continue cooking, uncovered, at a moderate boil for 5 minutes.

Add the sliced water chestnuts and scallion greens, poking them down into the liquid. Place the snow peas on top. Cover and return to a moderate boil. Uncover and adjust the heat to maintain a moderate boil for 3 to 4 minutes or until the snow peas are cooked thoroughly but still crunchy.

Move the chicken pieces to a platter with tongs. Skim the vegetables out with a slotted spoon and scatter them over the top.

Serve ½ to ⅔ cup of cooked rice in the bottom of each bowl. Divide the chicken and vegetables evenly among the bowls and top each with 1 cup broth.

SERVES 8

ROAST CHICKEN WITH ROASTED LEMONS AND WILTED WATERCRESS

Roasted lemons may sound odd, but they are very good—edible with a lovely flavor. SEE COLOR PLATE 3

> One 4½-pound chicken at room temperature, wing tips removed
>
> 6 lemons, each cut into 8 wedges, seeded, and the central membrane and thick peel tips cut away with scissors
>
> 2 tablespoons olive oil
>
> 2 large bunches watercress, arugula, or spinach, heavy stems removed (about 5 cups loosely packed)
>
> ½ cup chicken stock (any of the homemade stocks, pages 203–4, or sterile-pack)
>
> ¾ cups olives, such as Kalamata or Niçoise
>
> Kosher salt

Heat the oven to 500°F with a rack in the center. Place the chicken in a roasting pan no more than 2½ inches deep. Put in the oven legs first. Roast for 15 minutes. Take the pan from the oven and shut the door.

Jostle the chicken to unstick it. Rub the lemon pieces with the oil and place around the chicken in the pan. Return to the oven and roast for 10 minutes. Turn the lemon pieces over. Roast for 10 minutes more. Repeat. Carefully move the chicken to a platter, tilting it to allow any juices to run into the pan. Place the lemon pieces at one end of the platter.

Put the pan on top of the stove over high heat. Toss in the watercress. Stir-fry for about 4 minutes. Spoon the wilted leaves out onto the end of the platter opposite the lemons.

Return the pan to the heat. Add the chicken stock and olives. Cook until the olives are heated through. Add salt to taste. The amount will depend on the saltiness of the olives.

SERVES 2 TO 4 AS A MAIN COURSE

NAKED CHICKEN STEW

This is one of those put-your-money-where-your-mouth-is recipes. I opined on my blog that various foods were unnecessarily dredged (dressed) in flour before cooking. This recipe is proof positive. The end of the season vegetables from my garden gave all the body I wanted along with a freshness that the flour would have dimmed. I served it with corn fusilli (see page 39) in a deepish bowl with a spoon. It worked very well. For a thicker texture, use ¼ cup of cornstarch (see page 69 for basic instructions) at the end.

The quantities of vegetables can be approximated. This is a peasanty sort of dish.

> One 5-pound chicken, skinned and cut into parts, with breast cut across into 2 pieces (with optional addition of an extra breast cut into two or a leg and thigh, separated)
>
> 4 cups chicken stock (any of the homemade stocks, pages 203–4, or sterile-pack)
>
> 1 medium to large onion, cut into ¼-inch cubes
>
> ½ pound white mushrooms, cut into ¼-inch cubes
>
> 1 large or 2 medium tomatoes, cut into 1-inch cubes
>
> 3 medium bell peppers, preferably different colors, cored, seeded, and cut into ¼-inch pieces
>
> ¾ cup chopped basil
>
> ¾ cup finely chopped dill
>
> ¾ cup chopped parsley
>
> Kosher salt
>
> Freshly ground black pepper

Put the chicken pieces into a pot that holds them easily. Add the stock and enough water to barely cover. Bring to a boil. Reduce the heat to simmer. Add the onion, mushrooms, and tomatoes. Stir from time to time. After 20 minutes, add the peppers and basil. After 10 more minutes, add the dill and parsley. Cook for 5 minutes more. Season with salt and pepper to taste.

SERVES 4 TO 6

THE LADY IN RED

This is evidently based on coq au vin. However, cocks that require long cooking are hard to come by these days, as are hens. Instead this is adapted for a regular chicken. I think that you will find it rich enough to satisfy. Leftover wine or a half bottle should do nicely. Serve with gluten-free noodles, Garlic Mashed Potatoes (page 165), or Acorn Squash Purée (page 164). SEE COLOR PLATE 15

    1 pound smoky bacon in one piece, cut in half
    lengthwise and then across into ¼-inch strips

    One 5-pound chicken, skinned, cut into parts, with
    breast cut across into 2 pieces (with optional addition
    of an extra breast cut in two or a leg and thigh,
    separated)

    1¼ pounds white mushrooms, stems removed and
    sliced across, caps cut into quarters or sixths,
    depending on size

    1 pound cippoline or other small onions

    One 6-ounce can tomato paste

    ½ bottle red wine

    1 bay leaf

    2 cloves garlic, smashed and peeled

    ½ cup minced parsley

    1 teaspoon dried thyme

    Kosher salt

    Freshly ground black pepper

Put the bacon pieces in a pan just large enough to hold the chicken. Sauté the bacon until well browned and the fat has oozed out. Move the bacon to a small bowl, leaving the fat in the pan. Put the chicken pieces in the pan and sauté over medium heat, turning the pieces over from time to time, until lightly browned on all sides. Move to a bowl. Add the mushrooms to the pan and cook, stirring, until browned. Place in a bowl. Add the onions to the pan and cook until lightly browned. Move to the mushroom bowl.

Stir the tomato paste and wine into the pan. The sauce can be made ahead up to this point.

About 30 minutes before serving, add the chicken and bay leaf to the pan. Bring to a boil. Lower the heat and simmer for 30 minutes. Stick a knife into the thick part of the chicken to make sure it is done; the juices should run clear. Add the onions, mushrooms, and garlic. Cook until the vegetables are warm. Stir in the parsley and thyme and season with salt and pepper to taste. Stir in the bacon.

SERVES 4 TO 6 AMPLY

TANDOORI CHICKEN BREASTS

This mildly spicy version of a tandoori chicken—without skin—is easy. I keep most of the spices on hand. It is worth making an extra portion of the rub, which is also good on fish.

1½ tablespoons safflower oil

1 medium onion (about 3 ounces), cut into ¼-inch dice (1½ cups)

3 cloves garlic, smashed, peeled, and sliced across ⅛ inch thick

½ teaspoon ground cardamom

½ teaspoon cayenne pepper

⅓ teaspoon ground turmeric

¼ teaspoon ground cumin

¼ teaspoon ground mace

⅛ teaspoon dry mustard

⅛ teaspoon ground cinnamon

⅛ teaspoon freshly grated nutmeg

⅛ teaspoon freshly ground black pepper

1 teaspoon kosher salt

1½ teaspoons fresh lime juice

1½ tablespoons coconut milk

4 skinless and boneless chicken breasts (9 to 10 ounces each)

Heat 1 tablespoon of the oil in a large sauté pan over medium heat. When the oil shimmers, reduce the heat to low and add the onion, garlic, and all the spices, including the salt. Cook until the vegetables begin to turn translucent, about 10 minutes, stirring occasionally.

Using a spatula, move the contents of the pan to a blender. Add the lime juice and coconut milk. Blend well, about 1 minute. There will be ½ cup marinade.

Coat each chicken breast with marinade on both sides. Place the chicken breasts flat on a plate, cover with plastic wrap, and place in the refrigerator for 30 minutes. Heat the broiler with a rack in the middle.

Grease the bottom of a 10-×-8-×-1-inch pan with the remaining oil. Place the chicken breasts in an even layer in the pan. Broil for 10 minutes and then turn the chicken pieces over. Broil for 8 to 10 minutes longer. Remove from the oven and serve immediately.

SERVES 4

CHICKEN WITH CHERVIL SAUCE

Chervil is a pale green, frilly annual that sometimes comes back a second year and that is a dainty relative of parsley and lovage. Its tender leaves should be used raw, perhaps tossed into a salad, or exposed only briefly to heat. Its delicate flavor is like a cross between parsley and tarragon; longer cooking tends to turn it grassy. Chervil works particularly well with mild foods like poached chicken breasts, white-flesh fish, and eggs. Unlike other herbs, it is almost impossible to use too much.

To plant, sprinkle chervil seeds in partial shade every ten days during the summer to ensure a constant supply. Pick the outside leaves first. It can also be grown in a window box.

2 teaspoons vegetable oil

1 medium shallot, minced (3 tablespoons)

4 skinless and boneless chicken breast halves (about 1¼ pounds)

1¼ cups chicken stock (any of the homemade stocks, pages 203–4, or sterile-pack)

1 large bunch chervil leaves, all but 12 sprigs minced (about 3 tablespoons)

Kosher salt

2 tablespoons cornstarch

Heat the oil in a medium saucepan over low heat. Add the shallot and cook, stirring, for 3 minutes, until limp and translucent.

Add the chicken to the pan in one layer. Add the stock. Cover and bring to a boil. Turn the chicken over. Lower the heat, and simmer, covered, for 8 minutes. Add the minced chervil, turn the chicken again, and simmer, covered, for 4 minutes.

Remove the chicken and keep it warm. Season the broth with salt. Mix the cornstarch with 1 tablespoon water. Bring the broth to a boil. Pour the cornstarch mixture into the broth, whisking constantly. Return the sauce to a boil, still whisking. Lower the heat slightly and simmer for 2 minutes, whisking.

Serve the chicken with the sauce and sprigs of chervil.

SERVES 4

SPRING CHICKEN DELIGHT

I'm no spring chicken, but this recipe turns chicken into a spring treat with a plethora of only-in-the-spring vegetables. I prefer dark meat in this. It is cheaper than white and can take longer cooking and reheating; but if white is preferred, feel free.

I usually grill ramps on an outdoor grill, brushed with olive oil and the white part over the center of the heat and the greens off to one side. When I used the small amount of ramps that I had for this dish, it seemed sacrilegious to be cooking the ramp leaves; but it turned out very well.

I serve this chicken with grits (see page 221)—use polenta if it feels better.

> **2 tablespoons olive oil**
>
> **1¼ pounds young fennel, bulbs trimmed off, fronds reserved**
>
> **4 chicken legs and 4 chicken thighs (about 2½ pounds)**
>
> **½ pound ramps, green leaves cut across into 1½-inch pieces, white cut across into 2-inch pieces**
>
> **1 cup chicken stock (any of the homemade stocks, pages 203–4, or sterile-pack)**
>
> **10 ounces baby spinach**
>
> **Kosher salt**
>
> **Freshly ground black pepper**

Put the olive oil in a 4-quart braising pan (about 11 inches across). Warm it over low heat. While it warms, cut the fennel bulbs into wedges attached at the root end. They should be about ½ inch across at the base.

Raise the heat to medium and add the chicken pieces, skin side down. With tongs, move the pieces to keep them from sticking for 5 to 10 minutes and then turn the pieces on all sides until no red shows.

Pile the chicken pieces along one edge of the pot. Add the fennel wedges. Place the chicken pieces over the fennel so that there is a single layer of fennel. Cook for 10 minutes. Add the whites of the ramps. Stir, adding the chicken stock.

Raise the heat to simmer. Cook, scraping the bottom of the pot to incorporate any brown bits, for 10 minutes. Stir in the ramp greens and cook for 5 minutes. Stir in the spinach and cook for about 10 minutes or until the spinach is wilted. Add salt and pepper to taste.

SERVES 4 TO 8, DEPENDING ON APPETITES

NOT YOUR MOTHER'S COUSCOUS

Well, of course not, as couscous is a pasta made from wheat. I have adapted my recipe to use quinoa instead.

My first introduction to couscous was via Paula Wolfert's fabulous first book. This by no means implies that she is responsible for this recipe.

There is a little triumph hidden in this recipe, which is my substitute for classic preserved lemons. If you are one of those wonders who have preserved lemons on hand, you should certainly use them.

I put the almonds out in a bowl—some like them; some don't. Harissa is now readily available in markets. I find that which comes in tubes preferable.

If a good butcher is available, asking to have the chickens cut up as for Chinese stir-frying usually does the trick. Otherwise, use a good cleaver.

½ cup olive oil

1¾ pounds small onions (1½ to 2 inches across), stem and root ends removed (about 8 cups)

1 cup rice bran

One 4½-pound chicken, cut into about 16 small pieces through the bone

1 pound white mushrooms, stemmed and quartered (about 5 cups)

1½ pounds yellow bell peppers, cored, seeded, deribbed, and cut into 1-inch squares (6 to 7 cups)

1 head garlic, smashed, cloves separated, and peeled

2 cups unsweetened dried apricots

12 "Preserved" Lemon wedges (page 202)

Two 3-inch cinnamon sticks

2 tablespoons harissa

4 cups chicken stock (any of the homemade stocks, pages 203–4, or sterile-pack)

⅓ cup fresh lemon juice

Kosher salt

6 cups cooked quinoa (see page 168)

1½ cups whole roasted almonds

Heat the oil in a 6-quart braising pot over high heat. When the oil shimmers, add the onions. Cook until light brown, about 5 minutes, stirring occasionally. Move the onions to a platter.

Spread the rice bran on a newspaper or large sheet of parchment and dredge the chicken in it. Working in small batches (three or four pieces at a time), brown each piece of chicken in the hot oil, then move to a platter when done.

When finished browning the chicken, reduce the heat to low and return the onions and chicken to the pot. Add the mushrooms, yellow peppers, garlic, apricots, lemon wedges, cinnamon, and harissa. Pour in the chicken stock and stir to combine. Cover the pot and cook for 30 minutes. Remove the lid and simmer for 30 minutes more.

Season with the lemon juice and salt to taste. Serve with a bowl of quinoa and almonds on the side for people to add if they wish.

SERVES 4 TO 6

BASIC ROAST TURKEY

Aside from my recipe for roast chicken (see page 86) and perhaps a risotto or two, I don't think any recipe of mine has been reprinted, cooked from, and snared on the Internet more than this turkey.

I made it in honor of Thanksgiving on television on *Good Morning America*, where in her first forays into television Sara Moulton was the resident chef. Previously, she had worked for Julia Child. After the show, Julia called Sara and said: "Dear, they really should have said that the turkey was swapped for one that was cooked before." "No, Julia," Sara said. "It was cooked in real time."

Most of us live in real time; but we still want to eat well, and I think this is the best way to make a turkey. Cook the dressing (stuffing) separately. It's safer because it heats better without the bone shielding it. I do give stuffed roasting times for traditionalists.

If the turkey needs to be thawed, it will need a full day in the refrigerator. In any case, it will take several hours out on a counter to come to room temperature. Cover with a tent of foil or a damp cloth to keep the skin from drying out. I do not use store-bought turkeys that have been injected with stuff. I don't brine. High-heat roasted turkeys will stay moist from the melted fat under the skin. Wild turkey is too hard. There are very good heirloom birds.

See the timings at the right for different weights, unstuffed and stuffed. Be sure to save the carcass and bones from people's plates to make stock.

So here is my old friend one more time.

One 15-pound turkey, thawed if necessary and at room temperature, wing tips removed, giblets and neck reserved for gravy (see page 195), liver for dressing

Freshly ground black pepper

1 cup water or chicken stock (any of the homemade stocks, pages 203–4, or sterile-pack)

Heat the oven to 500°F with a rack on the second level from the bottom.

Rinse the turkey inside and out. Pat dry. Sprinkle the outside with pepper. If stuffing, stuff the cavity and crop (the neck skin), securing the openings with long metal skewers. Lace them. Do not truss.

Put the turkey in an 18-×-13-×-2-inch roasting pan, breast side up. Put in the oven legs first and roast for about 2 hours or until the leg joint near the backbone wiggles easily. After the first 20 minutes, move the turkey with a wooden spatula to prevent it from sticking. If it seems to be getting too dark, put a sheet of foil over the breast.

Move the turkey to a large platter and let sit for 20 minutes. Pour off or spoon out excess fat from the roasting pan and put the roasting pan on top of the stove. Add the stock and bring the contents of the pan to a boil while scraping the bottom vigorously with a wooden spoon. Let reduce by half. Serve on the side in a sauceboat or add to giblet gravy.

Basic Roast Turkey Times at 500°F

WEIGHT	UNSTUFFED	STUFFED
9 pounds	1 hour 15 minutes	1 hour 45 minutes
12 pounds	1 hour 20 minutes	1 hour 50 minutes
15 pounds	2 hours	2 hours 30 minutes
20 pounds	3 hours	3 hours 30 minutes

TURKEY AND CRANBERRY MEAT LOAF

I offer here a slightly sweet turkey and cranberry loaf baked in individual portions that children will find irresistible at Thanksgiving—or anytime. The fruit adds moisture, replacing the need for bread crumbs.

> ⅔ cup dried cranberries, coarsely chopped
>
> 4 very small stalks celery, peeled and cut into ¼-inch dice (⅔ cup)
>
> 1 medium bunch flat-leaf parsley, stemmed and finely chopped (⅓ cup)
>
> 1⅓ pounds ground turkey
>
> 1 scant tablespoon kosher salt
>
> 1 scant tablespoon celery seed
>
> 2 teaspoons dried sage
>
> 3 tablespoons vegetable oil
>
> Few grinds black pepper

Heat the oven to 350°F with a rack in the center.

Soak the chopped cranberries in ⅓ cup very hot tap water for 10 minutes; drain. Combine with all of the other ingredients.

Divide the mixture into four equal parts. Form into mounded ovals that do not touch and place in a 9-×-13-inch heatproof glass dish. Bake for 30 minutes. Let rest for 5 minutes. Using a pancake turner, transfer to individual plates and serve.

SERVES 4

A SINGLE SQUAB FOR THE HOLIDAYS

If you're alone at Thanksgiving or anytime, I suggest roasting a squab or a Cornish hen. Buy a can of cranberry sauce. Stick a sweet potato, its skin pricked with a fork, on a double sheet of paper towel in the microwave for 12 minutes. It will be done just before the squab. You're done. You can buy a tart.

> 1 medium squab (11 to 12 ounces)
>
> 1 tablespoon anise seeds
>
> ½ cup chicken stock (any of the homemade stocks, pages 203–4, or sterile-pack)
>
> Kosher salt
>
> Freshly ground black pepper

Heat the oven to 500°F with a rack on the second level from the bottom.

Put the bird in the smallest roasting pan available or on a pie plate. Put the anise seeds in the cavity. Place in the oven breast up, legs to the rear. Roast for 16 to 17 minutes. Move to a plate. Put the pan on the stove over high heat and bring to a boil with the stock and salt and pepper to taste. Scrape the pan and reduce liquid slightly. Eat.

SERVES 1

SQUAB WITH PEARS

Cooked and puréed Bosc pears make a pleasing and unusual sauce base for roast squab, a dark-meat bird that has only a hint of gamy flavor and can be served a little rare. Cornish hens, which taste more like chicken, are a good alternative. A 1-pound bird needs 15 minutes or so for roasting; larger hens will take longer and should be cooked until their juices run clear.

Buckwheat, with its mellow brown color, firm bite, and slightly nutty flavor, is a good contrast to the meat in this dish. Brown rice could be substituted but takes much longer to cook.

This is hearty food just right for an elegant winter dinner party. For a stunning presentation, I place the birds in a circle on a large round dish, put cooked pear halves between them, and mound the buckwheat in the center of the circle. I spoon a little pear sauce over each portion of bird and buckwheat; there will be enough left over for guests to add more if they wish.

½ cup chicken stock (any of the homemade stocks, pages 203–4, or sterile-pack)

¼ cup dry red wine

2 tablespoons red wine vinegar

3 firm ripe Bosc pears (about 1½ pounds), peeled, halved, and cored

1 cup buckwheat

4 medium squabs (11 to 12 ounces each), wing tips removed

2 tablespoons pear brandy (poire William)

Kosher salt

Freshly ground black pepper

1 tablespoon olive oil

½ teaspoon ground cardamom

2 to 3 scallions, trimmed and thinly sliced on the diagonal (½ cup)

Heat the oven to 500°F with a rack in the center.

In a saucepan just large enough to hold the pears in one layer, bring the chicken stock, red wine, and vinegar to a boil. Add the pears in one layer and simmer, covered, for 10 minutes, turning occasionally, until cooked through.

Cut two pear halves into chunks. Keep the remaining pears covered to keep them warm. In a blender, purée the chunks with the poaching liquid.

Bring 2 cups water to a boil. Add the buckwheat and return to the boil. Reduce the heat to simmer; cover the pan, and cook for 8 to 9 minutes.

While the buckwheat is cooking, rub each squab with pear brandy and sprinkle with salt and pepper. Place the squabs in a roasting pan and roast for 16 to 17 minutes or until the juices run clear.

Fluff the buckwheat with a fork and stir in the olive oil. Season with salt and pepper to taste.

When the squabs are roasted, remove to a platter. If the pears have cooled, reheat in the microwave for 2 minutes. Place the roasting pan on the stove over medium heat. Pour in ⅓ cup water and boil, scraping up any browned bits from the bottom of the pan with a wooden spoon. Stir in the pear purée and cardamom and bring to a boil. Season with salt and pepper and stir in the scallions. Spoon some sauce over the birds and buckwheat and pass the rest.

SERVES 4

ROAST QUAIL WITH FENNEL

I must confess that when I was in Syria I ordered and ate roast sparrows. They were delicious. At home, I do a similar thing with the equally small quail. The birds are often sold frozen, four to a package.

If they don't show up butterflied, cut along the length of the backbone with kitchen shears, open them out, and flatten them.

Teff (see page 169) would go well with this dish. SEE COLOR PLATE 16

> 1 large fennel bulb (1 pound), tops trimmed off, cut lengthwise through the core into ⅛-inch-thick slices so the core holds each slice in a whole piece
>
> 1 tablespoon olive oil
>
> ½ teaspoon kosher salt
>
> 2 teaspoons Lemon Zesty Spice Mix (page 202)
>
> 4 quails (3 to 4 ounces each), thawed if necessary and butterflied

Heat the oven to 500°F with a rack in the center.

Place the fennel slices in a 14-×-12-×-2-inch roasting pan. Drizzle the oil over the slices and turn until coated evenly. Arrange the slices in a single layer. Sprinkle with the salt. Roast for 10 minutes.

Rub the spice mixture over both sides of each quail. Set aside.

Remove the roasting pan from the oven and carefully turn the fennel with a spatula, pushing the pieces to the sides of the pan. Place the quails breast side up in the center aisle of the pan and roast for 5 minutes. Turn them over and roast for another 5 minutes.

SERVES 4 AS A FIRST COURSE, 2 AS A MAIN COURSE

ROAST DUCK WITH FORBIDDEN RICE

Dramatic, no? Forbidden rice is black rice that used to be restricted to royalty. Today, it comes in neat 1-pound packages and can be found on the Internet and in some groceries. Its deep flavor seems to be a perfect accompaniment for the richness of duck. Sadly, even though this dish is rich, one duck serves only four people.

My way of roasting duck is somewhat odd. It starts with poaching a duck whose skin has been thoroughly pricked so that the fat can ooze out. Then, it is roasted at high heat, making crisp skin and tender, juicy meat.

After the first go-round there will be duck stock on hand for future adventures, unless it has all gotten drunk in the meantime. If not drinking the stock, cook in it the reserved bones and innards—except the liver—and carcass of the duck, plus any bones that can be rescued from plates. Without duck stock, use chicken stock.

Fresh duck is preferable; but if frozen is all that is available, defrost it in the refrigerator overnight.

> 5½ quarts duck or chicken stock (any of the homemade stocks, pages 203–4, or sterile-pack)
>
> One 6-pound Long Island duck, thawed, giblets, innards, and wing tips removed and reserved, neck trimmed and reserved, and extra fat removed
>
> 4 teaspoons Lemon Zesty Spice Mix (page 202)
>
> 3 cups cooked black rice (see page 228)
>
> 1 bunch scallions, trimmed and cut across into ¼-inch slices (1½ cups)
>
> Kosher salt
>
> Freshly ground black pepper

Pour the stock into a tall narrow stockpot. Add the wing tips, neck, giblets, and any blood from the duck. Cover the pot and bring to a boil over high heat.

Meanwhile, using the tines of a fork, thoroughly prick the duck all over, paying special attention to the fattiest areas. Insert the tines at an angle so there is minimum risk of pricking the meat beneath. Carefully lower the duck into the boiling stock, neck end first. To keep the duck submerged, place a plate or pot over the duck to weigh it down.

When the stock returns to a boil, reduce the heat and simmer for 45 minutes. Check about every 10 to 15 minutes to see that the duck remains submerged. Keep the stock at a gentle simmer; if it boils, the duck will rise to the surface.

When the duck has finished simmering, spoon 2 tablespoons of the duck fat off the top of the stock and spread it in the bottom of a shallow 12-×-8-×-1½-inch roasting pan. Remove the plate and carefully lift out the duck, holding it over the pot to drain any liquid from the cavity. Place the duck in the roasting pan.

Leave the duck sitting out at room temperature to permit the skin to dry (the skin is very fragile at this point, so be careful) and heat the oven to 500°F with the oven rack on the second level from the bottom.

Sprinkle 2 teaspoons of the spice mixture all over the duck. Place the duck in the oven legs first. Roast for 30 minutes. After 10 minutes, pour out the fat that has accumulated in the roasting pan while carefully securing the duck. (Alternatively, gently remove the duck from the pan and pour the fat out, then return the duck to the roasting pan.) Move the duck around in the pan with a wooden spatula to prevent the skin from sticking to the bottom of the pan. In the meantime, skim the fat off the duck stock (there will be a lot).

When the duck has been roasting for 15 minutes, place the cooked black rice with a cup of duck stock in a medium saucepan over high heat. Bring the rice to a boil, reduce the heat to simmer, cook for 5 minutes, and add the sliced scallions. Once the rice is thoroughly warmed, turn the heat down.

After the full 30 minutes, remove the duck from the pan, allowing any interior juices to flow back into the pan. Put the duck on a serving platter. Pour or spoon off the fat from the roasting pan and place the pan on a burner over high heat. Deglaze with ½ cup duck stock. Season with salt and pepper to taste. Pour the gravy into a sauceboat.

Add the remaining 2 teaspoons spice mixture to the rice and turn the heat to medium, stirring well. If the rice appears dry, add more duck stock as needed. Spoon the rice into a serving bowl and serve with the duck.

SERVES 4

DUCK STEW WITH BLACK FIGS

The richness of duck has an affinity for young turnips in the spring. The figs are a good fall version.

Two 4-pound ducks, each cut into 16 serving pieces as for Chinese food (have the butcher do this), necks, gizzards, and wings reserved for stock

8 medium cloves garlic, smashed, peeled, and cut lengthwise in half

5 sage leaves

1 bay leaf

1½ cups medium-bodied red wine such as Rioja

32 small or 24 medium fresh black figs (1½ pounds), stemmed

1 tablespoon kosher salt, plus more to taste

Freshly ground black pepper

Heat the oven to 500°F with one rack in the bottom third of the oven and one in the top third.

With kitchen scissors, trim the excess fat from the duck pieces. Place the duck, skin side down, in one layer in two large heavy roasting pans. Roast for 15 minutes. Carefully remove the pans from the oven. Pour off the fat. Turn the duck meat side down. Return to the oven, placing the pan from the bottom rack on the top rack and vice versa. Roast for 15 minutes. Move the duck pieces to a bowl. Pour or spoon the fat from the pan. Reserve 2 tablespoons of the fat.

Place one pan on top of the stove. Pour ½ cup water into the pan. Bring the water to a boil, scraping any browned bits from the bottom and sides of the pan with a wooden spoon. Pour this liquid over the duck. Repeat with the second pan.

In a large wide pot, heat the 2 tablespoons reserved fat over medium heat. Stir in the garlic and cook, stirring, until the garlic is golden, about 4 minutes. With a slotted spoon, remove the garlic and add to the browned duck. Pour off the fat.

Put the duck with its liquid and the garlic in the pot. Add the sage, bay leaf, and 1 cup of the wine. Cover. Bring to a boil. Lower the heat and simmer gently for 45 minutes, turning the duck every 15 minutes.

Stir in the figs, salt, pepper, and remaining wine. Cover. Return to a boil. Lower the heat and simmer, 10 minutes for small figs, 10 to 15 minutes for medium. The figs should be cooked through while maintaining their shape.

Put the duck and figs on a serving platter. Pour the sauce into a measuring cup. Let the sauce sit for a minute or two, then skim the fat. Season with salt and pepper.

Serve the duck moistened with some of the sauce.

SERVES 6 TO 8

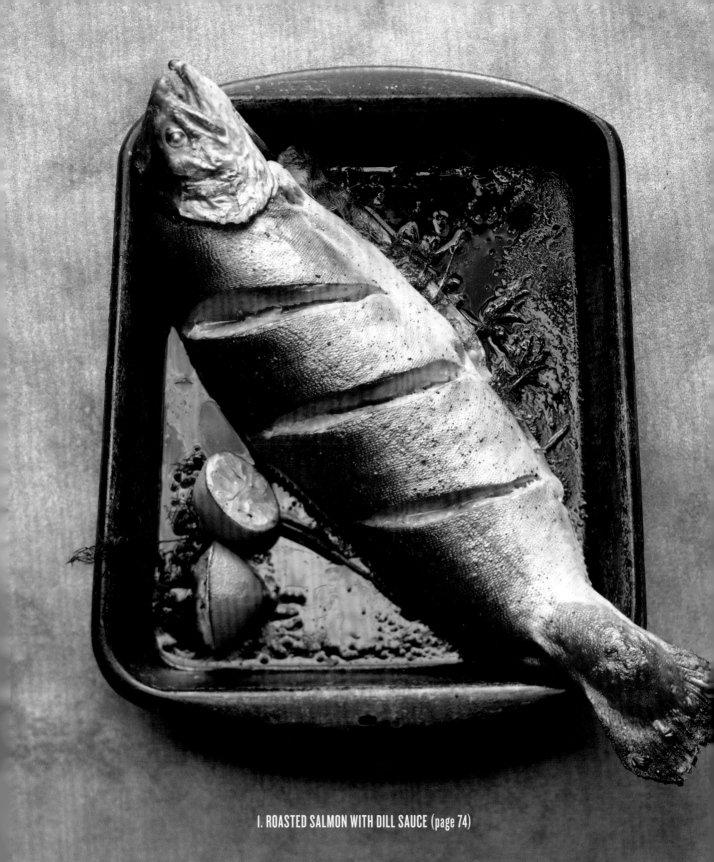

I. ROASTED SALMON WITH DILL SAUCE (page 74)

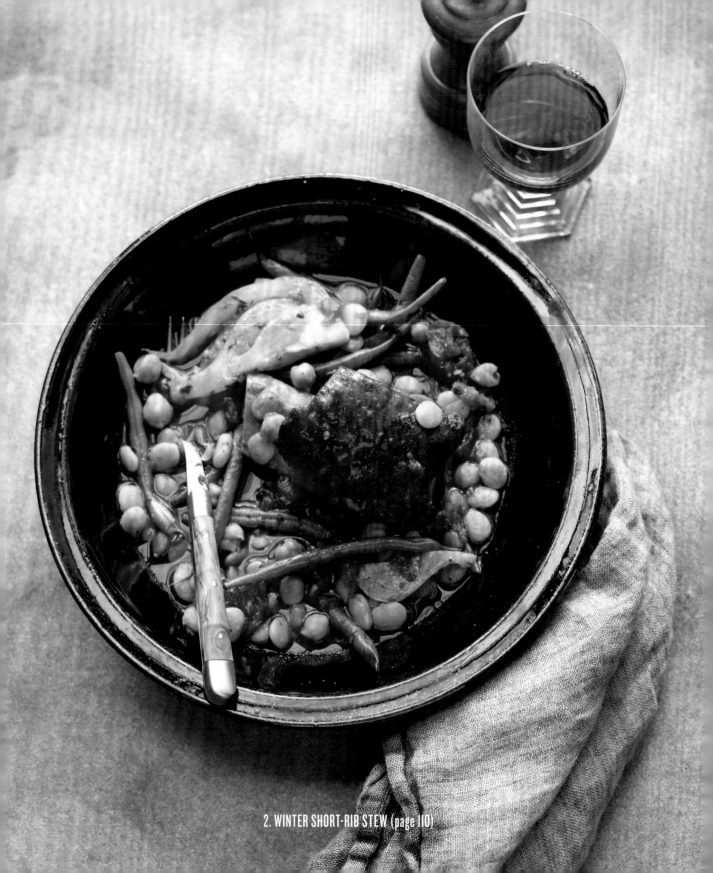

2. WINTER SHORT-RIB STEW (page 110)

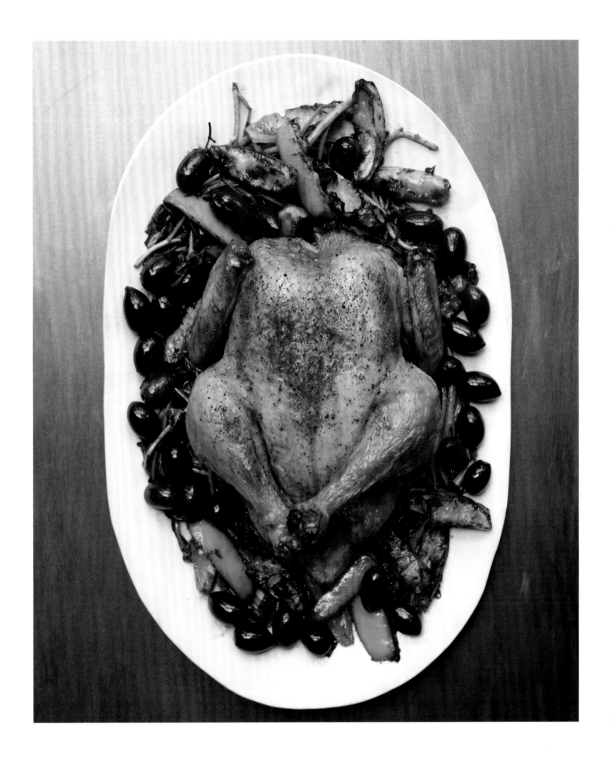

3. ROAST CHICKEN WITH ROASTED LEMONS AND WILTED WATERCRESS (page 89)

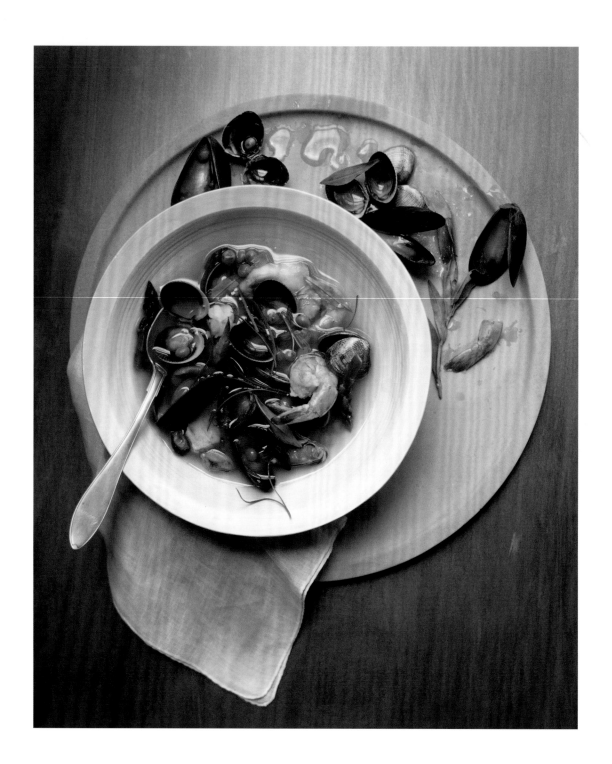

4. SPRING FISH SOUP (page 57)

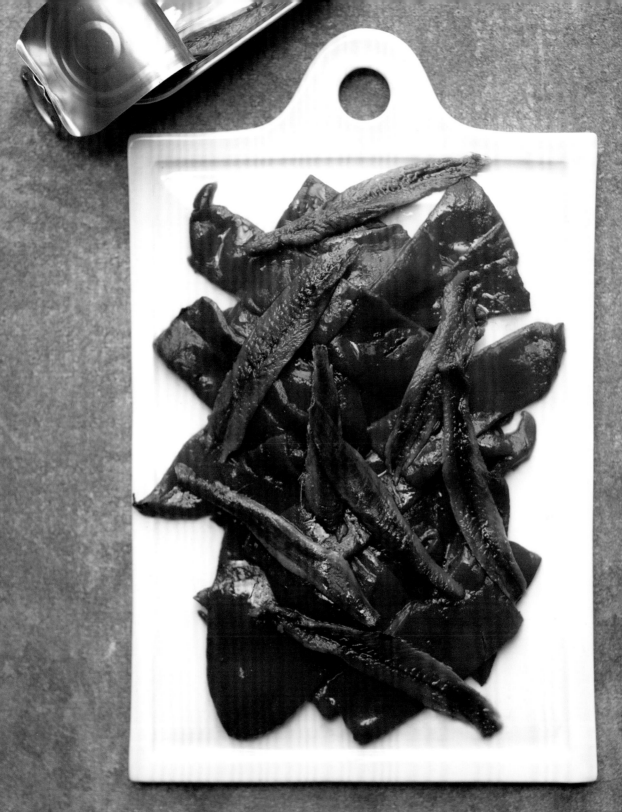

5. MARINATED PEPPERS (page 25)

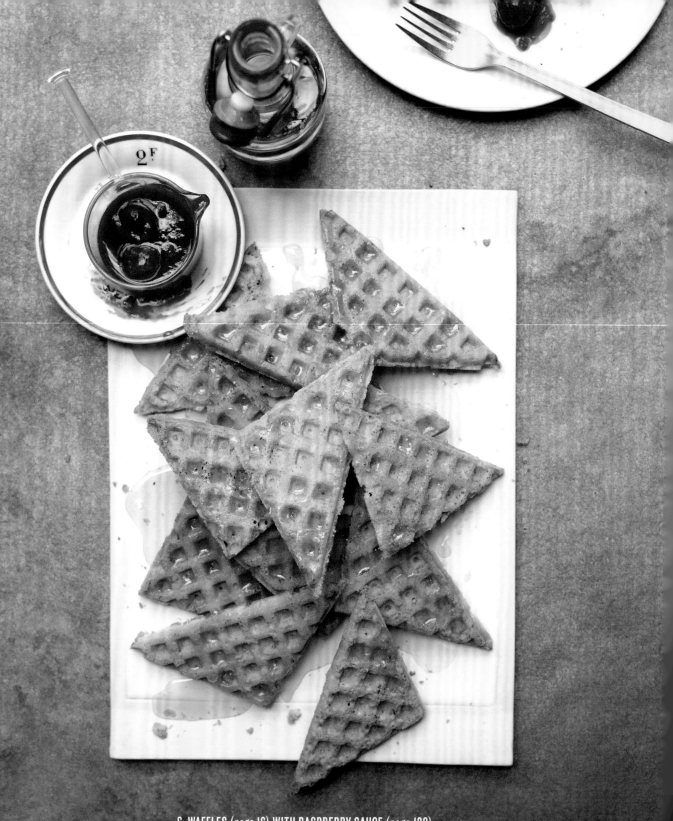

6. WAFFLES (page 16) WITH RASPBERRY SAUCE (page 199)

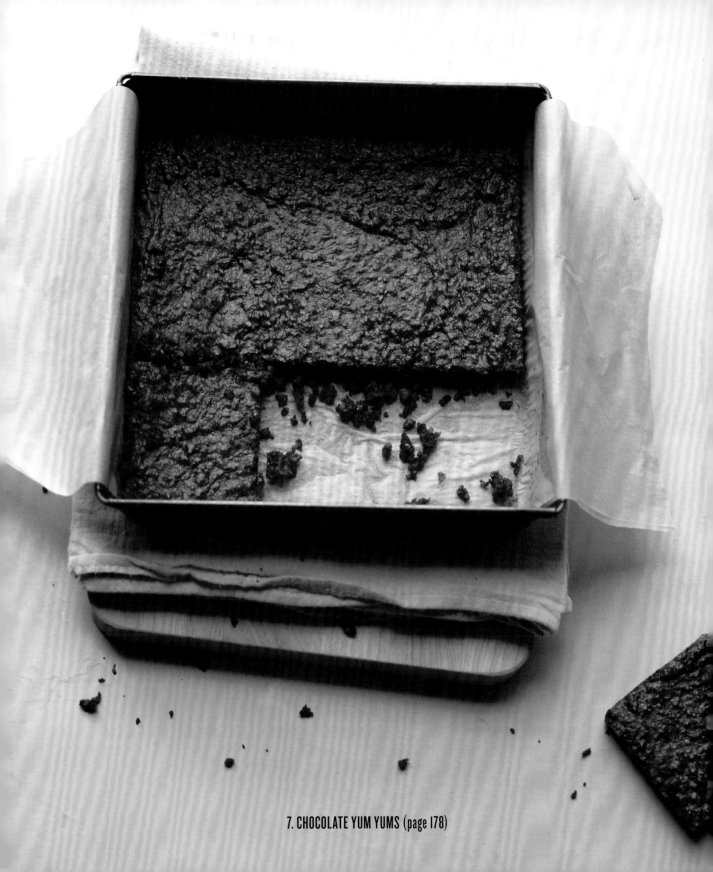

7. CHOCOLATE YUM YUMS (page 178)

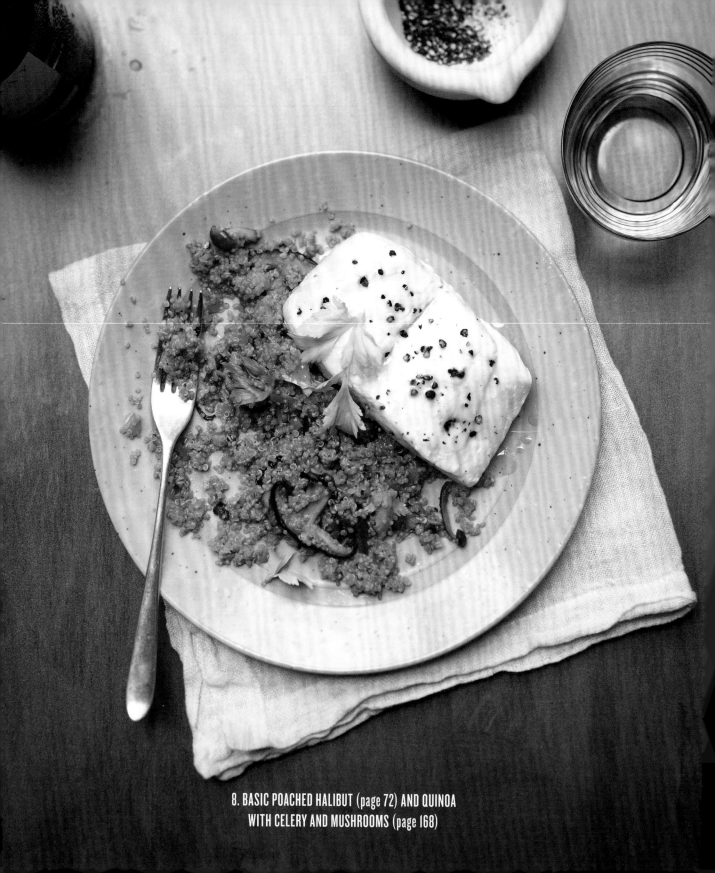

8. BASIC POACHED HALIBUT (page 72) AND QUINOA
WITH CELERY AND MUSHROOMS (page 168)

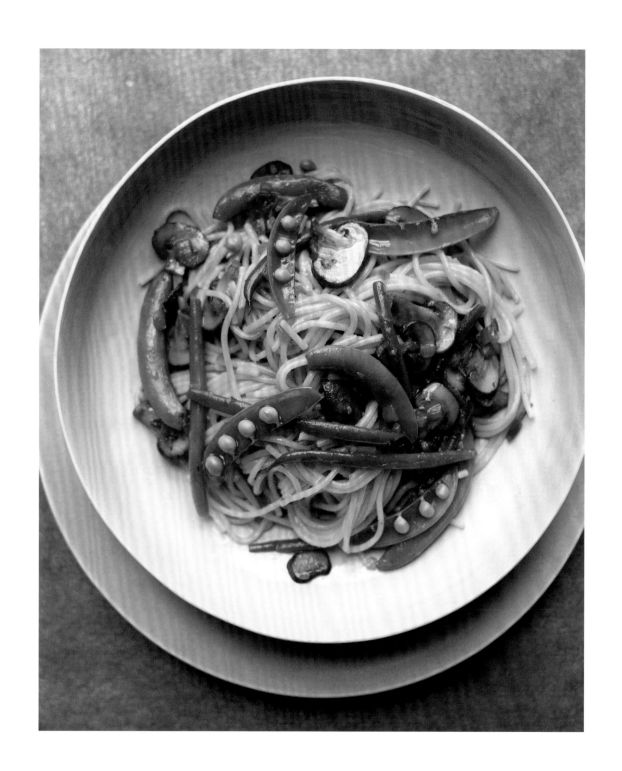

9. SIMPLE SPRING VEGETABLES WITH PASTA (page 146)

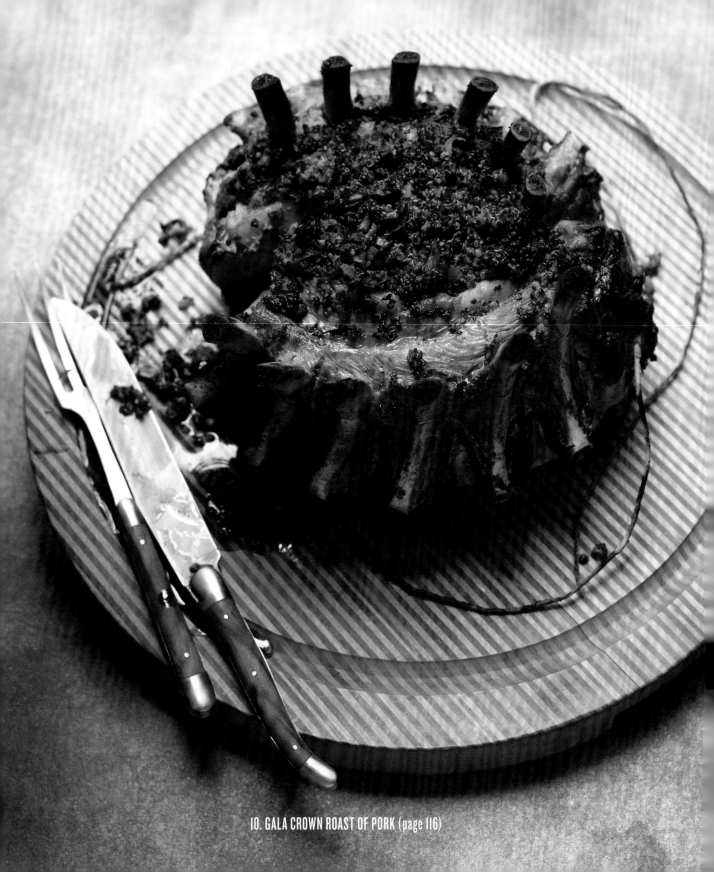

10. GALA CROWN ROAST OF PORK (page 116)

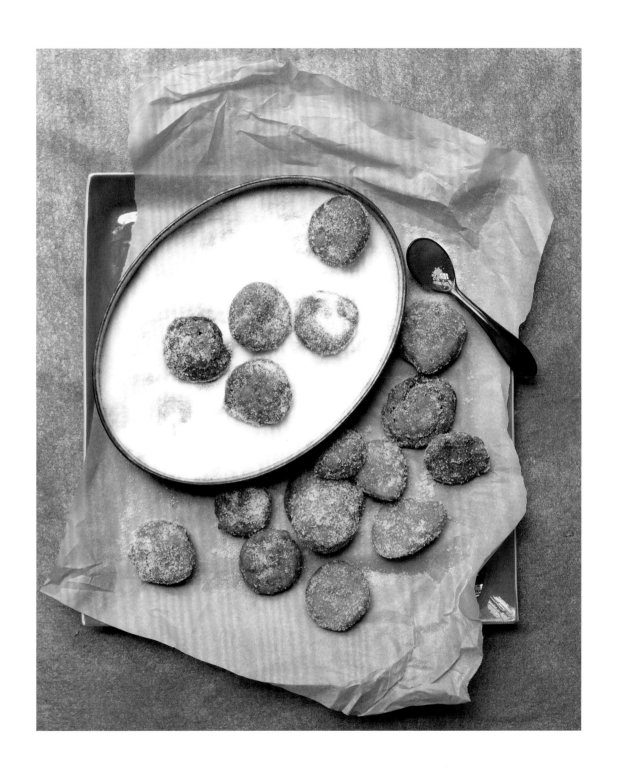

11. CHESTNUT DOUGHNUT HOLES (page 181)

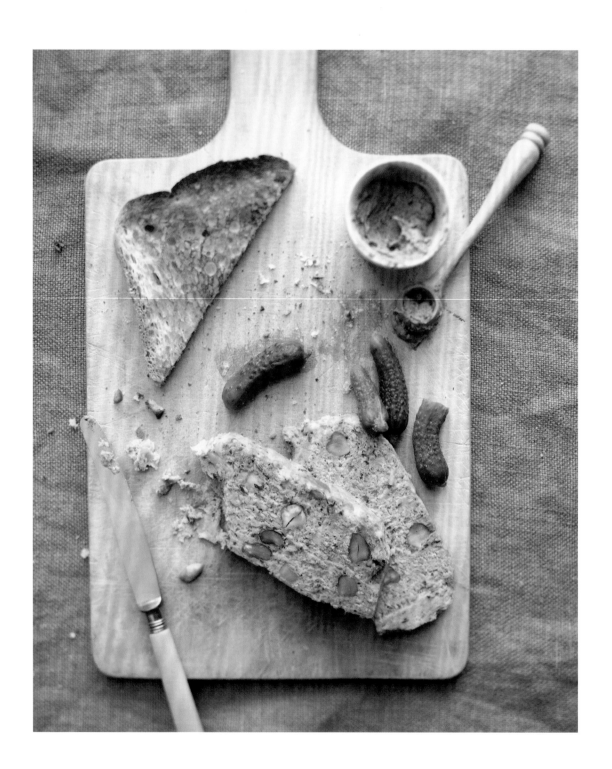

12. PORK-PISTACHIO PÂTÉ (page 31)

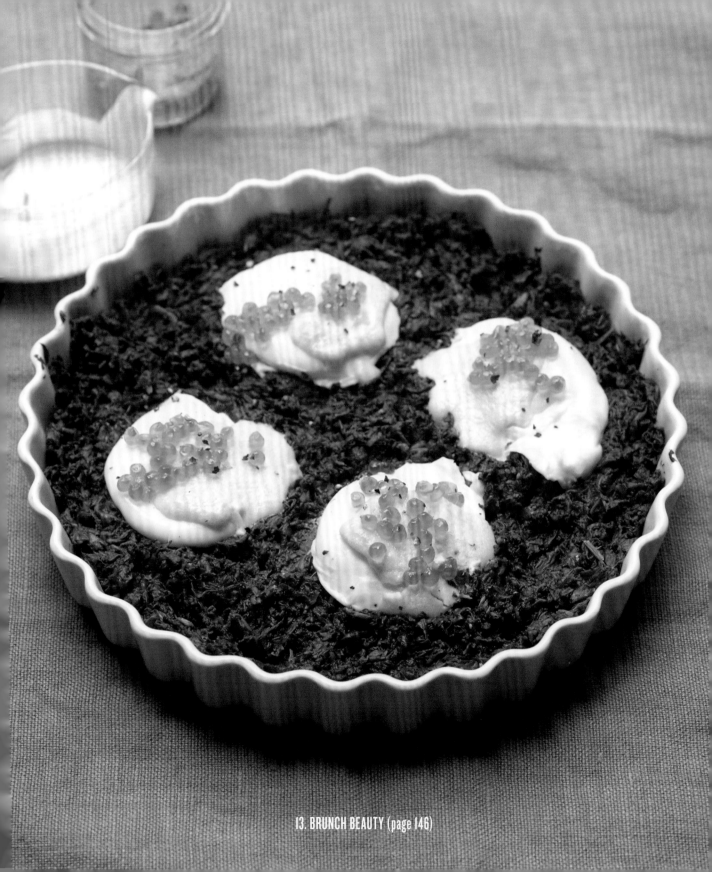

13. BRUNCH BEAUTY (page 146)

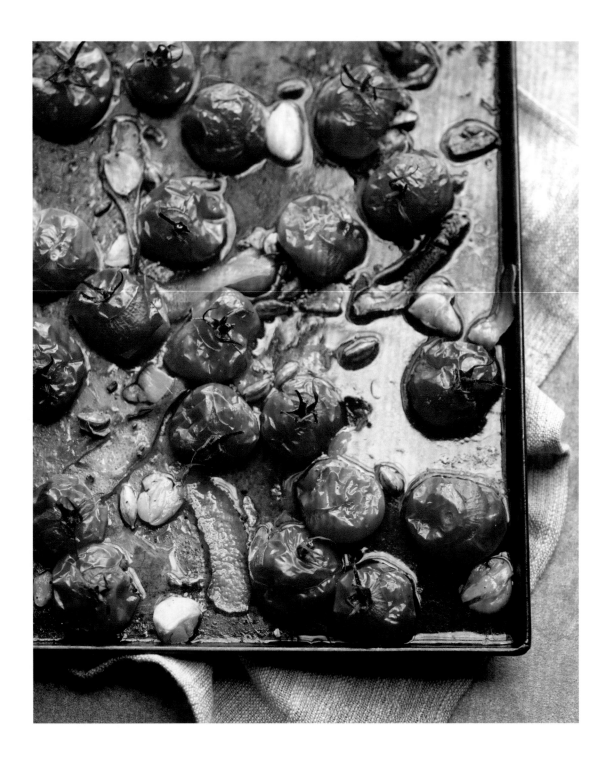

**14. ROASTED CHERRY TOMATOES WITH
ORANGE AND CARDAMOM (page 157)**

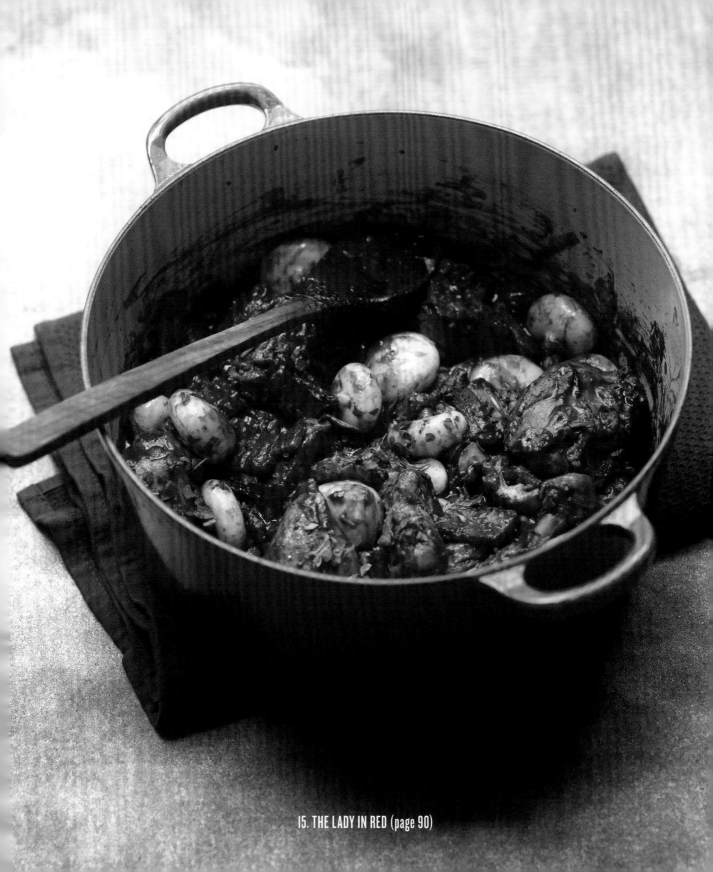

15. THE LADY IN RED (page 90)

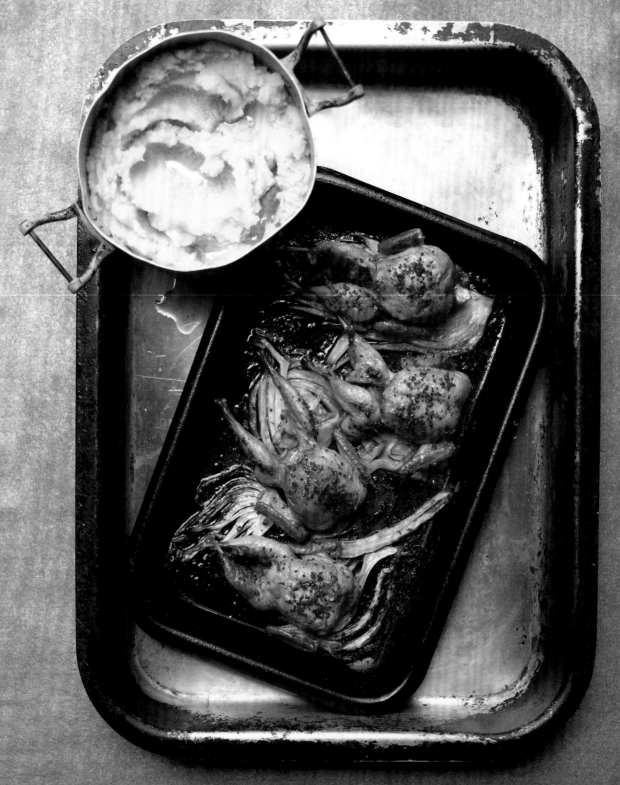

16. ROAST QUAIL WITH FENNEL (page 98) AND GARLIC MASHED POTATOES (page 165)

BEEF

Of course England has its Beefeater guards and its standing rib roast. However, if I were to define two countries as the home of beef, I would have to say Argentina and the United States. A great percentage of Argentine beef is sent to Europe and Africa as export products. Our beef stays at home and is a much beloved product.

By and large our beef is graded by the government, with prime at the top, followed by choice and good. There are two kinds of beef that are outside the system: Black Angus, mainly from Texas, and Wagyu and Kobe, Japanese breeds.

There is a dispute as to whether beef is best when grass fed or at least grass finished (fed on it toward the end of its life) or grain fed. There is little doubt any longer that organic beef without a load of hormones and other chemicals is better for us than nonorganic.

In general, beef should be aged. This doesn't mean old men. It means that once slaughtered, the beef should be hung in a temperature-controlled and well-aired space to develop flavor and soften. There are many debates over how long. At one time I worked for a brilliant restaurateur who earlier in his career used to go down to the—prefancy—Meatpacking District in Manhattan and mark the sides of beef that he selected with a special brand. Then they would be delivered at a date he designated.

The quality of beef is often designated by its marbling, which is the whitish threads and flecks of fat running through the red. As the meat cooks, the marbling melts, keeping the meat moist.

There are many cuts of beef. Consult your butcher or look at a good meat chart. Sadly, I cannot tell everything here. It should be noted that the tenderest cuts such as the tenderloin (filet mignon) do not have the most flavor and that some of the slightly chewier cuts such as the sirloin and hanging tender have the most flavor. Ground beef for ham-burger offers a choice of round and chuck. Round will have less fat and less flavor than chuck.

LUXURY BOILED BEEF

Luxury boiled beef is derived from a very elegant French dish, *boeuf à la ficelle*, in which a whole filet of beef wrapped in a cloth is simmered in broth. This quick version is elegant enough for any dinner party and is made with very quickly cooked slices of filet mignon. The meat flavors the broth along with the vegetables, especially the leek and tarragon.

The starch—gluten-free pasta noodles or Olive Oil Mashed Potatoes—can be served right in the soup since there are no bones to worry about.

> 5 small carrots, peeled and cut into ⅛-×-⅛-×-1½-inch strips
>
> 1 medium leek, white and light green part only, cut into ⅛-×-⅛-×-1½-inch strips and then soaked in water for 10 minutes to remove grit
>
> ½ pound haricots verts (slim green beans), tipped and tailed
>
> 6 ounces fresh shiitake mushrooms, stemmed and cut across into ¼-inch-thick strips
>
> 8 cups chicken stock (any of the homemade stocks, pages 203–4, or sterile-pack)
>
> Six 1-inch-thick slices filet mignon (2 pounds)
>
> ¼ cup loosely packed tarragon leaves, plus about 18 leaves for garnish
>
> 1 tablespoon kosher salt
>
> Freshly ground black pepper
>
> 3 cups gluten-free pasta noodles (see page 39) or Olive Oil Mashed Potatoes (page 165)

Place the vegetables in the bottom of a large wide-mouthed pot. Toss to combine. Add the stock. Cover and bring to a boil. Uncover, reduce the heat, and cook at a medium boil for 5 minutes.

Add the meat in one layer on top of the vegetables. Poke the meat down into the liquid so that all the pieces are covered. Cover. Turn the heat up slightly to maintain a moderate boil. Cook for 5 minutes.

Move the meat to a platter. Stir the tarragon, salt, and pepper to taste into the soup.

Use ½ cup noodles or mashed potatoes per person. If using a large wide-rimmed soup bowl, place the noodles in the bowl and top each with a piece of filet mignon, a cup of broth, and just under a cup of vegetables. Garnish with a few leaves of tarragon.

SERVES 6

GRILLED FLANK STEAK

Of course this can easily be broiled as well. If grilling, see page 11 for basics.

Flank steak isn't the tenderest piece of meat, but I am very fond of it. Briefly cooked to sear on both sides, rare, and sliced correctly, it is delicious.

To slice, start in one corner and, with the blade of the knife at about a thirty-degree angle to the board or platter and about ¼ inch in, start to cut the meat thinly—about ¼ inch thick—into slices. Proceed down the steak until the opposite corner is reached.

1 flank steak (about 1¾ pounds)
2 teaspoons kosher salt
Freshly ground black pepper
½ cup olive oil

Sprinkle both sides of the steak with the salt and pepper to taste. Coat with the oil and allow to stand at room temperature for at least an hour, turning at least once.

Preheat a grill until the coals are white-hot. Grill the meat for about 10 minutes on each side for medium-rare, depending on the heat of your grill.

Remove the meat from the grill and allow to stand for about 5 minutes before slicing.

SERVES 5 OR 6

SPINACH MEAT LOAF

Fresh, homemade meals can actually be convenient—as long as they're not fancy or show-offy. This meat loaf, too, cooks handsomely in the microwave in less than 20 minutes.

1 pound spinach, stemmed
1 medium onion (6 ounces), peeled and quartered
3 cloves garlic, smashed and peeled
¾ cup cooked quinoa (see page 168)
¼ cup plus 1½ teaspoons teff flour
½ cup plus 1 tablespoon ketchup
2 tablespoons gluten-free soy sauce
Freshly ground black pepper to taste
1½ pounds lean ground beef, preferably top round

Place the spinach in a 10-inch pie plate or quiche dish. Cook, uncovered, on high for 5 minutes in a microwave oven. Remove from the oven and let stand until cool.

Place the spinach in a food processor and coarsely chop. Put in a large mixing bowl. Place the onion and garlic in the food processor and finely chop. Add to the spinach along with the remaining ingredients except the beef and blend well. Once the mixture is uniform, add the beef and combine well.

Transfer the mixture to a 9-×-5-×-3-inch glass loaf pan, making sure there are no air pockets. Cover tightly with microwave-safe plastic wrap and cook on high for 15 minutes. Prick the plastic to release steam.

Remove from the oven and uncover. Cover with a kitchen towel and let stand for 15 minutes. Serve hot or cold.

SERVES 4 TO 6

SAUTÉED BEEF WITH PEPPERS, ONIONS, AND MUSHROOMS

This simple sauté makes the delicious most out of a small amount of an expensive cut of beef. Serve with rice or rice noodles. Those who like spicier food can add the chili oil.

I like to make this in a wok, which makes the stir-frying easier.

¾ pound beef tenderloin (filet)

¼ cup safflower oil

1 large onion, cut in half and then across into ¼-inch half-moons (about 2 cups)

4 or 5 large white mushrooms, stemmed and cut into ¼-inch slices (about 1½ cups)

1 large green bell pepper, cored, seeded, deribbed, halved lengthwise, and cut into ¼-inch slices (about 2 cups)

⅓ cup Worcestershire sauce

2 tablespoons potato starch

1 tablespoon toasted sesame oil

1 tablespoon sesame seeds

2 tablespoons chicken stock (any of the homemade stocks, pages 203–4, or sterile-pack)

1 teaspoon chili oil (optional)

Slice the beef across into ⅛-inch-thick slices. If using the tail end of the tenderloin, be sure to slice at a severe diagonal to make larger slices of meat. If using the thicker portion of the tenderloin, make sure to pound the slices of meat with the flat side of the blade if they are too thick. Place the slices evenly on a plate and set aside.

Pour the oil into a wok over high heat. When the oil shimmers, add the onion. Stir-fry until the onion is translucent, about 3 minutes. Add the mushrooms and green pepper. Cook, tossing, for 3 to 4 minutes more. Add the beef, piece by piece (to prevent sticking), cooking and tossing just until the beef is done, 1 to 2 minutes.

Whisk the Worcestershire sauce and potato starch together and pour into the beef and vegetable mixture. Combine well (the mixture will get thicker). Turn off the heat. Add the sesame oil, sesame seeds, stock, and chili oil, if using.

SERVES 4

SIMPLE RIB ROAST

My roast is rare, but no Saxon pillage. The outside slices can serve the meat eaters who like it better done. The technique and timings are simple. First, the meat is roasted for three-quarters of an hour at 500°F, then for approximately 3 minutes per pound at moderate heat, and finally, the roast is hit with high heat for another 15 minutes. Plan on 1 hour and 12 minutes for a small roast and 2 hours and 15 minutes for a large one.

If the consensus of friends is for the meat to be "bloody, bawdy," I take the 3 minutes a pound down to 2. If they want it medium, the 3 minutes goes to 5. For well done, heaven help them. These times presuppose the meat at room temperature and at least 15 minutes of sitting time after the meat comes from the oven, when it will continue to cook.

One 4½-pound short (without short ribs) standing rib roast (2 ribs) or one 26-pound standing rib roast (7 ribs total)

2 to 6 cloves garlic, smashed, peeled, and slivered (optional)

Kosher salt

Freshly ground black pepper

½ to 2½ cups red wine for deglazing

Heat the oven to 500°F with a rack on the second level from the bottom.

Place the small roast in a 14-×-12-×-2-inch roasting pan, bone side down; the large roast will need an 18-×-13-inch roasting pan. Snuggle most of the garlic under the fat and spread the remainder under the meat. Season the roast well with salt and pepper. Roast for 45 minutes. Reduce the heat to 325°F and roast for another 12 minutes for the small roast, for another 1 hour and 15 minutes for the large roast. Increase the heat to 450°F and roast for 15 minutes more for either size. An instant-read thermometer should reach 135°F.

Remove the roast from the oven. Move to a serving platter. Pour or spoon off excess fat, reserving about ⅛ cup fat for the small roast and ¼ cup fat for the large roast. Put the pan over high heat with the reserved fat and add the wine. Deglaze the pan well, scraping with a wooden spoon. Let reduce by half. Pour the liquid into a small sauceboat and serve with the roast.

SMALL ROAST SERVES 2 TO 4; LARGE ROAST SERVES 10 TO 12

MEXICANISH OXTAILS

While I was in Mexico, I went into a huge supermarket. There were the products that I was used to as well as Mexican staples. I used ingredients that I usually don't. The bouillon cubes eliminated the need for extra liquid. The only thing to keep in mind is that the oxtails will have to be ordered ahead and ensuing negotiations take place with the butcher to slice them.

Serve this over rice.

¼ cup olive oil

2 oxtails (about 8 pounds), cut into 1-inch-thick slices

2 medium onions, thinly sliced

2½ cups red wine, plus more to taste

3 cups tomato purée (homemade, page 208, or sterile-pack)

5 cloves garlic, smashed and peeled

6 Knorr chicken bouillon cubes

Kosher salt

Freshly ground black pepper

4 to 5 mild hot peppers such as jalapeños

2 teaspoons dried oregano

I use two 12-inch sauté pans to accelerate the process, but, of course, the cooking can be done in batches. Place 1 to 2 tablespoons oil (per batch) into a sauté pan over high heat. Sear the oxtail pieces in a single layer until browned. Turn over. Continue cooking in batches until all the pieces are browned.

Put the oxtails in a casserole or a Dutch oven. Put the onion slices into the remaining fat and brown lightly; add to the meat. Pour in the wine and add the tomato purée. Tuck in the garlic cloves and bouillon cubes. Sprinkle with salt and pepper to taste. Put the jalapeños on top with the oregano. Cover. Cook over medium heat for 2½ to 3 hours, until the meat is soft. Add more red wine if desired.

SERVES 6 TO 8

ROAST BEEF HASH

The word "hash" comes from the French *hacher*, which means "to chop." Curiously, though, the French do not make hash as we know it: the dish seems to have developed in countries where beef and leftover potatoes were plentiful. Ireland comes to mind.

Whatever. It all starts with a boiled potato. The best potatoes for hash are the floury kind suitable for mashing, like russets from Idaho and Maine. To cook them, cut in half and cover them with water in a medium saucepan. Bring the water to a boil, lower the heat slightly, and cook for 20 to 25 minutes, until the potatoes are tender.

3 tablespoons olive oil

1 medium onion, chopped

1 pound floury potatoes, cooked, peeled, cooled, and cut into ¾-inch cubes

2 pounds rare cooked roast beef (such as from Simple Rib Roast, page 108), cut into ¾-inch cubes

1 cup chicken stock (any of the homemade stocks, pages 203–4, or sterile-pack) or beef stock

6 ounces spinach leaves, blanched and squeezed dry

¼ cup chopped parsley

½ teaspoon chopped thyme or a pinch dried

½ teaspoon chopped sage or a pinch dried

Kosher salt

Freshly ground black pepper

Add the oil to a large nonstick skillet over medium heat. Stir in the onion and cook, stirring occasionally, for 6 minutes.

Heat the broiler. Stir the potatoes, roast beef, and stock into the onion. Cook, stirring, until the mixture is fairly dry. Stir in the spinach, herbs, and salt and pepper to taste. Cook, stirring, until everything is well mixed and hot.

Turn out into an ovenproof dish and brown under the broiler.

SERVES 4

WINTER SHORT-RIB STEW

Short ribs, normally served solo, can be converted into a fine stew too, with or without the bones.

The secret to stews lies in the thickening, the same element that sets a braise apart from a brothy soup. Stews may contain more solids, or the savory liquid in which they cook may be thickened. Either way, there is that satisfying density.

Many times the thickening is added at the beginning of a stew, but it can also be added toward the end of cooking via a paste of cornstarch and cold water, called a "slurry." But there are sneakier ways. Puréed, cooked, or canned chickpeas will also act as a thickener—and provide a boost of nutrition. SEE COLOR PLATE 2

3 pounds short ribs, cut across and between the bones to form 12 pieces about 2 inches square (see Note)

6 cloves garlic, smashed and peeled

3 cups diced canned or sterile-pack tomatoes

1 bay leaf

Four 1-×-4-inch strips orange zest

One 1-×-3-inch strip lemon zest

1 pound thin green beans, tipped and tailed

2 tablespoons kosher salt, or to taste

1 large bulb fennel, stalks removed, cut in half, cored, and cut into thin strips

1 tablespoon coarsely chopped oregano

1 tablespoon coarsely chopped thyme

One 10-ounce package frozen baby lima beans, defrosted in a sieve under warm running water

¾ cup canned chickpeas, drained and rinsed

Freshly ground black pepper

Heat the oven to 500°F with a rack in the center.

Place the short ribs in one layer in a medium roasting pan and roast for 25 minutes. Turn the pieces, add the garlic, and roast for 15 minutes more.

Put the ribs into a tall, narrow stockpot. Spoon off the fat from the roasting pan and pour any juices over the bones.

Place the roasting pan on top of the stove over medium heat and add 1½ cups water. Bring to a boil, scraping any browned bits off the bottom of the pan with a wooden spoon. Pour this liquid over the bones.

Add the tomatoes, 2 cups water, the bay leaf, two pieces of the orange zest, and the lemon zest. Cover the stockpot and bring to a boil. Uncover, lower the heat, and simmer for 40 minutes.

Stir in the green beans and 2 cups water. Cover and bring to a boil. Uncover, lower the heat, and simmer for 30 minutes, occasionally poking the beans down into the liquid. Add 2 teaspoons of the salt and simmer for 10 minutes.

Skim the fat. Add the fennel and the herbs. Bring to a boil. Lower the heat and simmer for 5 minutes. Add the remaining salt, the lima beans, chickpeas, remaining two strips of orange zest, and 2 cups water.

Bring to a boil, lower the heat, and simmer for 5 minutes. The meat should be falling off the bones. Season with pepper to taste.

Remove the meat and the bones from the stockpot. Place two pieces of meat (with or without the bones) in each of six bowls and divide the vegetables and liquid evenly over them.

MAKES 6 HEARTY SERVINGS

NOTE

Have the butcher do the cross-cutting. If the short ribs are cut in overlarge sections, there will be fewer than 12 pieces. If so, cook them as described and remove the meat from the bones before dividing it evenly among the bowls.

BEEF DAUBE

Daube is a traditional dish from the South of France. There is even a special pot for it called a *daubière,* earthenware and rounded toward the bottom to accommodate all the solids, with a narrower neck that causes the liquid fat to rise so that it is more easily skimmed off. It has a lid.

Pastis and Pernod are anise-flavored liquors also native to southern France. If unavailable, use Cognac.

¼ cup olive oil

3 pounds boneless beef chuck, cut into palm-size, ½-inch-thick slices

2 yellow onions (about 1¼ pounds), cut in half, then across into thin slices

¼ cup pastis, Pernod, or Cognac

2 oranges, 5 strips zest removed with a potato peeler, then juiced (about ⅔ cup)

⅔ cup red or white wine

1 cup chicken stock (any of the homemade stocks, pages 203–4, or sterile-pack) or beef stock

1½ tablespoons tomato paste

One 4-×-4-inch square pork rind or 3 thick strips lean bacon

Large pinch dried savory

Large pinch dried sage

Large pinch dried marjoram

2 bay leaves

1½ ounces garlic, smashed and peeled, half left whole, half chopped

4 sprigs thyme

¾ cup olives, preferably picholine or Niçoise

One 2-ounce tin oil-packed anchovies, drained and chopped

2 tablespoons drained capers, rinsed

Preheat the oven to 325°F with a rack in the bottom third.

Heat the oil in a large skillet until smoking. Add as many pieces of beef as will fit in a single layer. Cook until browned, turning once. Move to a plate. Repeat with the remaining pieces.

Pour or spoon off half the fat. Stir in the onions. Cook until nicely browned. Remove. Pour or spoon off the remaining fat. Add the liquor. Warm gently and flame. Allow the flames to die down. Add the orange juice, wine, stock, and any meat juices on the plate. Deglaze the pan, scraping up the brown bits. Stir in the tomato paste. Remove from the heat.

Put the pork rind or bacon, skin side down, inside the bottom of a 3-quart casserole dish, preferably stoneware or earthenware, with a lid. Layer ingredients into the dish, starting with the meat. Continue layering with the onions, savory, sage, marjoram, and bay leaves. Sneak the whole garlic cloves in among the layers. Push the thyme and orange zest into the center.

Pour the deglazing liquid on top. Cover with the lid and bake for 2½ hours. Check to see if the meat is tender. If not, continue cooking until it is.

Remove the thyme sprigs. Put the meat in a bowl or serving dish. If feeling very French, cut the pork skin into small bits and add to the meat; otherwise, discard it. Remove the bay leaves. Pour the cooking liquid into a saucepan. Skim off the fat. Add the olives. Bring to a boil. Allow to cook over low heat until the olives are hot.

Mix in the chopped garlic, anchovies, and capers. Return the meat to the cooking pot if attractive. Otherwise, pour the sauce over the meat in a serving dish.

SERVES 8

A SLOW BEEF MELT

Rump roast is a chewy piece of meat, but it makes up for that in flavor. I have had a Crock-Pot for years but almost never used it. Some kind person sent me a rice cooker thinking, I suppose, that it could compensate for the loss of noodles in my diet. I almost always cook rice the way I have for years, but I discovered the virtues of the rice cooker as a slow cooker for meat and beans. Its temperatures are much more stable than those of the old Crock-Pot, and it heats up more quickly. I was elated and went out and bought a large slow cooker that can do large cuts of meat.

Yes, my kitchen looks like Fibber McGee and Molly's, but it is worth it.

This slow-cooked rump roast—two sizes—is not just like a braise or a pot roast. It has a purity of flavor that is very seductive. The meat gives off a great deal of liquid, and I put a soup bowl next to each meat plate, with a spoon, of course.

This dish takes about half a day to cook, but actual prep time is minimal and the results are well worth the wait. Enjoy this hearty dish with a side of boiled potatoes (Yukon Gold work quite nicely), a bowl of quinoa (see page 168), or, if you're feeling generous, both. The choice of mushrooms will determine the ultimate cost.

One 3-pound chunk beef rump

1 medium unpeeled onion

½ lemon, juiced, keeping the rind

1½ cups chicken stock (any of the homemade stocks, pages 203–4, or sterile-pack)

1½ cups red wine

½ pound white mushrooms, trimmed and cut into ¼-inch slices, or 1 pint fresh morels, rinsed

½ bunch oregano, chopped (about 2 tablespoons)

1 bunch parsley, chopped medium fine (about 1 cup)

Kosher salt

Freshly ground black pepper

Place the beef, unpeeled onion, lemon juice and rind, stock, and wine in a slow cooker. Make sure the onion is covered with liquid; if not, cut the onion into quarters. The liquid should come about a third of the way up the pot. Cook on the lowest setting for 6 to 6½ hours or until the meat is very tender. About 30 minutes before the end of the cooking, add the mushrooms. After the meat is done, switch off the power and turn the meat over to even out the color.

Remove the meat and mushrooms to a platter and discard the lemon rind. Reserve half the liquid in a separate pot. Squish the onion out of its skin by pressing on it with a fork (it should slide right out) and discard the skin; if the onion is in quarters, peel away the skin and throw it away. Mash the onion with the fork until it dissolves into the cooking liquid in the original pot. Pour the reserved liquid into a large saucepan. Reduce the volume by half over medium-high heat. Add the herbs (see Note) and season to taste with salt and pepper. To serve, slice the beef and surround it with the mushrooms. Put the reduced liquid into a bowl and serve with a ladle.

SERVES 4 OR 5

NOTE

If serving with quinoa, add the chopped herbs to it instead of the beef.

VARIATION

This recipe can easily be doubled by using a 6-pound rump, 2 whole onions, 1 whole lemon, 3 cups chicken stock, 3 cups red wine, 1 pound sliced mushrooms or 2 pints fresh morels, ¼ cup chopped oregano, and 2 cups chopped parsley. It will serve 8 to 10 people.

PERFECT PIG

This name might describe me as well as the title of this chapter. I love every aspect of pork, "including the squeak," as the saying goes. Be careful about sausages as well as all other prepared foods; they may well contain wheat flour or bread as a binder. The other parts of the pig not found in this chapter will be in "Other Meats" (page 136).

GALA CROWN ROAST OF PORK

The ingredients alone make this a gala dish, but it is not all money and show. It is delicious. It goes very well with steamed broccoli. SEE COLOR PLATE 10

> 1 full crown roast of pork, chine bone removed, bones frenched, bones at spine end cut apart to facilitate carving (done by a good butcher)
>
> ¼ pound dried morels, preferably small
>
> 1 ounce dried porcini
>
> ⅔ ounce dried oyster mushroom slices
>
> 1 tablespoon olive oil
>
> ¼ pound yellow onion, cut into ¼-inch dice (about ⅔ cup)
>
> ⅓ cup loosely packed finely chopped flat-leaf parsley
>
> 1 tablespoon chopped sage
>
> 1 tablespoon kosher salt
>
> Lots of freshly ground black pepper
>
> 1½ cups cooked quinoa (see page 168)
>
> ½ teaspoon caraway seeds

Carefully check the inside of the roast. Remember that the inside of the circle is the side of the roast normally on the outside. With a sharp pointed knife, remove as much extra fat as possible from the inside. If the butcher has not already done it, make little wrappings of aluminum foil to cover the exposed top bones. Place the roast in a pan large enough to hold it comfortably.

Boil 2 cups water. Add the morels and cook for 2 minutes. Remove from the heat. Remove the morels with a slotted spoon and reserve. Line a sieve with a damp tea towel. Pour the morel liquid through the cloth or a coffee filter.

Return the liquid to the pot with enough water to make 4 cups. Bring to a boil and add the porcini and oyster mushroom slices. Boil for 2 minutes. Remove with a slotted spoon and reserve.

Heat the oven to 500°F with a rack on the second level from the bottom.

Meanwhile, cook the liquid in the pot to reduce to ¾ cup.

Heat the oil in a small sauté pan over medium-low heat. Cook the onion until soft and translucent, about 10 minutes. Coarsely chop the porcini and oyster mushrooms and any large or mushy or torn morels. Toss with the onion, herbs, salt and pepper, quinoa, caraway seeds, and ¼ cup of the reduced mushroom liquid.

Grease a 6-inch square of aluminum foil. Pile as much of the stuffing into the center of the crown roast as possible, patting it down and mounding it. Reserve any extra stuffing. Cover the stuffing with the greased foil. Put the roast in the oven for 50 minutes. Remove the foil. Roast for 15 minutes more. Check the temperature of the meat with an instant-read thermometer, making sure the tip isn't touching bone and goes toward the center into the thickest part. If the temperature has not reached 145°F, return the roast to the oven until it has.

Remove the roast from the oven. Either with a strong commercial hamburger spatula or with hands and two clean kitchen towels, move the roast to a platter. Remove the foil from the bones.

Put the pan on top of the stove. Add the remaining ½ cup reduced mushroom liquid, 1½ cups water, and any leftover stuffing. Bring to a boil, scraping the bottom of the pan to dissolve all the meat juices.

Serve the roast carved into chops with a large spoonful of dressing and pass the deglazing liquid as a sauce.

In addition to your carving knife and fork, be sure to have kitchen scissors on hand as string will have been used to form the crown.

SERVES 9

NEW ROAST PORK

This is a new version of one of my old favorites, boned and rolled loin of pork. It looks and tastes sensational.

1 teaspoon dried marjoram

1 teaspoon dried sage, crumbled

2 teaspoons kosher salt

⅛ teaspoon freshly ground black pepper

One 3-pound boneless pork loin, bones reserved if available

2 pounds cippoline or other small onions, peeled and root ends trimmed

Heat the oven to 500°F with a rack in the center.

Combine the marjoram, sage, 1 teaspoon of the salt, and the pepper in a shallow dish large enough for the pork to lie flat. Roll the pork loin in the spice mix until well crusted. Place in a roasting pan, along with the reserved bones toward one side.

Roast for 20 minutes. Add the onions to the pan, turning them in the liquid. Season with the remaining salt. Roast for 30 minutes longer.

Remove the pan from the oven and transfer the roast, bones, and onions to a platter. Deglaze the pan (see page 12) with ¼ cup water and drizzle the sauce around the food.

SERVES 6 NORMAL PEOPLE OR 4 OF MANY OF MY FRIENDS

ROAST PORK TENDERLOIN WITH BARBARA'S FIVE-SPICE POWDER

Well, I made the powder for sweet treats, but I found myself licking my fingers and thinking of all the things on which it would be good. There are other recipes in the book that use this powder; but this was the first, which came out of the oven for dinner yesterday—good too. The tenderloins come two to a package. One would probably be a slightly skimpy amount for four, but two would be good for six. I served it with the Quinoa with Celery and Mushrooms (page 168) and sautéed spinach (see page 18). Soup first and berries for dessert.

If the tenderloins are frozen, refrigerate them overnight and then allow them to come to room temperature.

2 teaspoons olive oil

Two 1-pound pork tenderloins (each about 10 inches long and 2½ inches in diameter)

2 tablespoons Barbara's Five-Spice Powder (page 202)

Heat the oven to 500°F with a rack on the second level from the bottom.

Rub the bottom of a 12-x-8-x-1½-inch roasting pan with the oil. Rub each tenderloin with 1 tablespoon of spice mixture. Let rest in the pan side by side—not touching—for about 20 minutes. Roast for 10 minutes. Turn each tenderloin over. Roast for 10 minutes more.

Move the tenderloins to a serving platter. Pour off any fat in the pan. Place over high heat. Add ½ cup water, boil, and scrape to deglaze. Cut the tenderloins into 1½-inch-thick slices on the diagonal.

SERVES 4 TO 6

SOY-MARINATED PORK SHOULDER

This makes a delicious small roast with an Asian flair. Start it well ahead of roasting—even the night before—to let the meat absorb the flavors.

> 1 cup gluten-free soy sauce
>
> ½ cup rice vinegar
>
> 1 teaspoon grated ginger (¾-inch piece of peeled ginger)
>
> 1 teaspoon minced garlic (1 to 2 small cloves)
>
> 2 tablespoons plus 2 teaspoons brown sugar
>
> 12 drops Tabasco sauce
>
> 1½ pounds boneless pork shoulder
>
> 1 to 2 teaspoons safflower oil

Combine all the ingredients except the pork and oil in a small saucepan over medium heat and stir until the sugar dissolves, 2 to 3 minutes. Pour the marinade into a medium bowl and allow to cool. Place the pork in the bowl and cover directly with a paper towel (the towel will absorb the marinade and make sure the meat never dries out on top). Cover the bowl with plastic wrap and refrigerate overnight.

A few hours before roasting, take the bowl out of the refrigerator.

Heat the oven to 500°F with a rack on the second level from the bottom.

Spread the oil evenly on the bottom of a shallow 12-×-8-inch roasting pan. Shake the excess marinade from the pork and place the roast in the center of the pan.

Roast the pork for 20 minutes. Reduce the heat to 450°F and roast for 40 minutes longer, until the internal temperature reaches 160°F on an instant-read thermometer. Remove the pork from the oven and let it rest for 10 minutes. Slice and serve.

SERVES 4

SOY-MARINATED PORK SHOULDER
HORS D'OEUVRE

When we made this, I liked it so much that I thought it would make a great munch with drinks. It does. It can also be a main course.

> 1 cup gluten-free soy sauce
>
> ½ cup rice vinegar
>
> 1 teaspoon grated ginger (¾-inch piece of peeled ginger)
>
> 1 teaspoon minced garlic (1 to 2 small cloves)
>
> 2 tablespoons plus 2 teaspoons brown sugar
>
> 12 drops Tabasco sauce
>
> 1 pound boneless pork shoulder or pork chops, trimmed of visible fat, bones removed, and cut into 1-inch cubes
>
> 1 to 2 teaspoons safflower oil

Combine all the ingredients except the pork and oil in a small saucepan over medium heat and stir until the sugar dissolves, 2 to 3 minutes. Pour the marinade into a medium bowl and allow to cool. Place the pork in the bowl, cover with plastic wrap, and marinate for 1 hour. Place fifteen to seventeen 4-inch wooden skewers in a bowl and cover with water.

Heat the broiler with the oven rack in the top level. Spread the oil evenly on the bottom of a shallow 12-×-8-inch roasting pan. Place two pork cubes 1 inch apart on each skewer. Spread the skewers out evenly on the greased roasting pan and broil for 3 minutes. Remove from the oven and allow to rest for 2 to 3 minutes. Serve hot.

MAKES 15 TO 17 SKEWERS; SERVES 4 AS A MAIN COURSE

ETUDE NUMBER THREE
SOY-MARINATED PORK SHOULDER

This version of the marinated pork shoulder is fancy enough for a party. Remarkably, the tomatoes keep their shape despite the long cooking time. The roast requires a large slow cooker. The natural sauce will be a happy addition to cooked quinoa (see page 168), teff (see page 169), or Garlic Mashed Potatoes (page 165).

1⅓ cups gluten-free soy sauce

⅔ cup rice vinegar

1½ teaspoons grated ginger
(1-inch piece of peeled ginger)

1½ teaspoons minced garlic (1 to 2 cloves)

3 tablespoons brown sugar

Several drops Tabasco sauce

2 pounds boneless pork shoulder

1½ pounds (4 to 5) small tomatoes

6 cloves garlic, smashed and peeled

2 bay leaves

2 tablespoons plus 2 teaspoons olive oil

10½ ounces white mushrooms, stemmed and sliced
¼ inch thick (5 to 6 cups)

1½ tablespoons fermented black beans

Combine the soy sauce, vinegar, ginger, garlic, brown sugar, and Tabasco in a small saucepan over medium heat and stir until the sugar dissolves, 2 to 3 minutes. Pour the marinade into a medium bowl and allow to cool. Place the pork in the bowl and cover directly with a paper towel (the towel will absorb the marinade and make sure the meat never dries out on top). Cover the bowl with plastic wrap and refrigerate overnight or for 6 hours at cool room temperature.

Place the pork in a slow cooker and pour all the marinade over it. Add the tomatoes, garlic, and bay leaves. Cook for 1 hour on high, then reduce the heat to low and cook for 5 hours more.

Pour the olive oil into a 10-inch sauté pan over high heat. Add the mushrooms and cook until tender, 3 to 4 minutes. Thirty minutes before the pork is done, add the mushrooms and black beans to the slow cooker. When the pork is finished cooking, slice and serve.

SERVES 4

PORCINE VICTORY

It is amazing how small victories can delight a cook. The other day I had bought a pork chop to serve at dinner. I was admonished that, while my pork roast was delicious and really hefty pork chops came out okay, regular pork chops tended to be dry and tough. I chewed on that for a while and decided there had to be a solution.

It is ironic that as our pork has been bred to be leaner and leaner we are being told that rare breeds—of great price—are to be prized for their fat content. It is of course that fat that kept the meat moist and tender. However, the new, leaner pork is better for us. I cogitated and am delighted to have come up with a solution.

This recipe can be multiplied to make as many chops as there are eaters as long as the sauté pan is large enough to hold them in a single layer.

1 teaspoon toasted sesame oil

1 rib pork chop (about ½ pound)

1 ounce peeled ginger, coarsely grated (1 tablespoon)

2 cloves garlic, peeled, smashed, and thinly sliced across

2 tablespoons gluten-free soy sauce

¼ teaspoon Chinese five-spice powder

¼ pound small tomatoes, cherry or any other shape

Put the sesame oil into a 9-inch pan over medium heat. Put in the pork chop. Cook, turning once, until white on both sides. Put the ginger and garlic around the edges. Pour the soy over all. Sprinkle with the five-spice powder. Surround the chop with the tomatoes. Cover and simmer for 15 minutes or until white throughout.

SERVES 1

ROAST PORK LOIN WITH TURNIPS

This dish would be very good served alongside some green beans, which also love sage.

One 2½- to 3½-pound boneless pork loin (8 to 10 inches long), bones reserved, if available

4 cloves garlic, smashed, peeled, and cut lengthwise into thin slivers

10 sage leaves, rolled and cut across into thin strips

Kosher salt

Freshly ground black pepper

6 large turnips (about 2 pounds), trimmed, peeled, and cut into 6 wedges each

½ cup red wine for deglazing

Heat the oven to 500°F with a rack in the center.

With the point of a paring knife, make ½-inch slits toward the center all around the roast. Insert the garlic in the slits, accompanied by a few strips of sage. Rub the roast generously with salt and pepper.

Place the roast and bones in a roasting pan large enough to hold them surrounded later by the turnips. Roast for 5 minutes. Surround with turnip wedges in one layer. Roast for 15 minutes. Turn the wedges over. Roast for 15 minutes more. Turn the wedges again and roast for 15 minutes or until the meat reaches an internal temperature of 140°F. The meat might still be slightly pink. Don't overcook the roast or it will be dry and unappealing.

Move the roast and bones to a platter. Surround with the turnips. Let the meat rest before slicing across, while preparing the sauce. Snip off the strings. The juices will collect better in a platter than on a cutting board.

Place the pan on top of the stove over high heat. Add the wine and bring to a boil. Stir in the remaining sage. Scrape the pan with a wooden spoon to remove the glaze that will flavor the sauce. Cook until reduced by half. Serve in a sauceboat or a bowl along with the roast.

MAKES 10 GENEROUS SLICES; SERVES 6 TO 8

AROMATIC PORK IN COLD VEGETABLE SAUCE

Like many cooks, I often shy away from cooking meat on a hot summer's night—unless someone else volunteers to fire up the grill, of course. But roasts and other large cuts of meat do not have to be forsaken completely when it's hot outside: simply poach them ahead of time and serve them cool, with a flavorful sauce on top. With a salad on the side, you've got an easy supper that cuts down on heat in the kitchen and gives the cook a well-deserved break.

This aromatic pork is accompanied by its very own sauce, which is made by puréeing the vegetables the pork cooks with and then adding a small amount of olive oil. (Be sure to ask your butcher to give you the bones after the pork loin has been boned, because they will add flavor to the sauce.)

Also be sure to turn the pork in the pot so that it cooks evenly.

2 pounds onions, quartered

¾ pound carrots, peeled and cut across into 1-inch pieces

¾ pound celery, peeled and cut across into 1-inch pieces

¼ cup sage leaves

2 cloves

6 medium cloves garlic, smashed and peeled

2 tablespoons kosher salt

2 pounds boneless pork loin, rolled and tied, bones reserved, if available

2 tablespoons olive oil

In a 10½-inch-wide braising pan or stockpot, bring 14 cups water to a boil with the onions, carrots, celery, sage, cloves, garlic, 1 tablespoon of the salt, and the pork bones. Add the pork loin, pushing it down into the pot until it is covered with water. Return to a boil. Lower the heat and simmer for 30 minutes. Turn the pork and simmer for another 30 minutes. Turn the pork and simmer for 15 minutes more or until a meat thermometer inserted in the center of the loin registers 145°F.

Remove the pot from the stove and allow the meat to cool in the liquid. Move the meat to a platter. With a slotted spoon, scoop the vegetables from the pot. In a food processor, purée the vegetables with the remaining salt and the olive oil; there should be about 6 cups of sauce.

Slice the meat across into ¼-inch-thick slices; there should be about two dozen slices in all.

Spread a cup of sauce on a medium platter or in a baking dish. Place a layer of pork slices on top of the sauce and then spread the slices with more sauce. Continue until all the sauce and meat have been used. Cover with plastic wrap and refrigerate for 1 hour or up to 3 days.

SERVES 6

CLARA'S PEACHY KEEN PORK CHOPS

This may read like an oddity. Instead, it is a sensational summer supper that is also easy to prepare and lovely to look at with its soft colors. This recipe can easily be doubled or halved. The pork chops taste even better the next day, after being drenched in sauce all night.

Make extra sauce. It is also good on chicken and fish.

CLARA'S PEACHY KEEN SAUCE

    2 peaches (6 ounces each)

    1 tablespoon safflower oil

    2 cloves garlic, smashed , peeled, and chopped

    ½ small onion, roughly chopped (about ¼ cup)

    ¼ cup ketchup

    1½ tablespoons sherry vinegar

PORK CHOPS

    1 tablespoon safflower oil

    Two 1½-inch-thick pork chops (¾ pound each)

    Kosher salt

    Freshly ground black pepper

    5¼ cups Soft Polenta (page 170)

Heat the oven to 450°F.

MAKE THE SAUCE: Place the peaches directly on a burner over high heat and char on all sides, 2 to 3 minutes. Remove the peaches from the heat, place in a bowl, and cover tightly with plastic wrap.

Pour the oil into a 10-inch skillet over medium heat. Sauté the garlic and onion until soft, 2 to 3 minutes. Remove the skin and flesh from the peaches, discarding the pits, and put in the pan, breaking up larger pieces with a wooden spoon. Add the ketchup, vinegar, and ¼ cup water and simmer over medium-low heat until the peaches are fully cooked and most of the water has evaporated, about

5 minutes. Using a spatula, scrape the contents of the pan into a food processor and blend until the mixture is smooth and of uniform consistency, about 4 minutes. Set the sauce aside.

COOK THE PORK CHOPS: Heat the oil in an ovenproof 10-inch skillet over high heat. Season the pork chops with salt and pepper. When the oil shimmers, gently place the pork chops in the pan. Brown the pork chops for 2 minutes, turn over, and brown for 1 minute. Place the pan in the oven and bake the chops for 8 to 10 minutes. Take the pan out of the oven, remove the pork chops to a plate, and let rest for at least 5 minutes.

Warm the polenta in the microwave for 2 minutes and then spread on a large platter. Slice the pork chops off the bone into ¼-inch slices and fan out on top of the polenta. Pour the sauce generously over the pork.

SERVES 4

SPIFFY SPICE PORK CHOPS

I recently made pork chops for dinner and wanted to do something special. I made this very simple spice mixture and have since found it good for chicken and large mushrooms as well. It serves as a replacement for breading and browns well. The mixture can be multiplied and kept tightly sealed to use as desired.

SPIFFY SPICE MIXTURE

2 tablespoons Chinese five-spice powder

1 tablespoon ground cumin

PORK CHOPS

2 extra-thick rib pork chops (about 1 pound each)

1 tablespoon olive or safflower oil

¼ cup tequila

1 tablespoon kosher salt

Freshly ground black pepper

MAKE THE SPICE MIXTURE: Combine the spice mix ingredients in a pie dish or flat plate. Lay the pork chops on top and turn several times to coat thoroughly.

COOK THE PORK CHOPS: Heat the oil in a heavy sauté pan just large enough to hold the chops next to each other over medium-high heat. Put in the chops. Brown on each side for 5 to 6 minutes. Cover and turn the heat down to medium. Cook for 12 minutes. Toward the end of the chop cooking time, put the tequila in the smallest saucepan available and heat. Pour off the fat from the chops. Carefully, with a match, flame the tequila and pour it over the chops. Allow to cook until the flames die. Season with the salt and pepper to taste.

SERVES 2

HAM AND SWEET POTATO HASH

Traditionally hash, the quintessential comfort food, has been the perfect answer for leftovers—as long as they included an ample supply of boiled potatoes and some sort of meat.

The ham and sweet potato hash here, adapted from a recipe by James Villas, can use leftover ingredients from a holiday dinner if you have them (if you don't, just go for it anyway). The potatoes add an element of sweetness, and the ham gives the dish a homey, particularly American touch.

¾ pound cooked lean ham, cut into ¼-inch dice

1 pound sweet potatoes, cooked, peeled, and cut into ½-inch dice

1 small onion, cut into small dice

½ medium green bell pepper, cored, seeded, deribbed, and cut into small dice

3 eggs

1 tablespoon chopped fresh sage or 1 teaspoon dried

Freshly ground black pepper

3 tablespoons safflower oil

In a large bowl combine the ham, sweet potatoes, onion, and green pepper. In a small bowl, whisk together the eggs, sage, and pepper to taste and add to the ham mixture.

Heat the broiler.

Add 1½ tablespoons of the oil to a medium skillet over high heat. When the oil shimmers, add the ham hash, reduce the heat to medium, and cook for 4 minutes, gently shaking the pan occasionally to loosen the bits at the bottom.

To brown the top, invert the hash into an ovenproof dish, drizzle with the remaining oil, and place under the broiler for 3 to 5 minutes.

SERVES 4

PORK WITH GREEN FIGS AND APPLES

Whether a luscious purple or a pearly light green, figs are always a special treat. Their somewhat mysterious, deep taste can be emphasized by cooking and can add a gentle, unexpected richness to meaty stews as well as desserts.

The pork stew uses pale green figs, which give the dish a pale color. In this country the green figs are likely to be Kadota, which most of us see dried. They are excellent fresh, however, with lighter meats and desserts.

Green apples add a welcome note of acidity and crispness. I serve this with white rice.

1 tablespoon safflower oil

2 pounds boneless pork loin, cut into 1-inch pieces

1 medium yellow onion, cut into ¼-inch dice

2 tablespoons Dijon mustard

10 medium green figs (about 1 pound), stemmed

2 medium tart green apples, like Granny Smith, peeled and cut into ¼-inch dice

Juice of 1 lemon

2 tablespoons kosher salt, or to taste

2 tablespoons cornstarch

Freshly ground black pepper

In a medium saucepan, heat the oil over medium-high heat until shimmering. Working in batches, brown the pork, about 1½ minutes per side. As each batch is done, set it aside in a bowl. When the last batch has browned on one side, turn the pork and stir in the onion. Continue to cook, stirring, until the onion is slightly softened and brown, about 5 minutes. Stir in the mustard and then scrape the mixture into the bowl with the rest of the browned pork.

Lower the heat slightly and place the figs in the bottom of the saucepan. Toss the apples in the lemon juice and then sprinkle the apples over the figs. Return the pork and onion to the pan.

Add 1 cup water and sprinkle with 1 teaspoon of the salt. Cover. Bring to a boil. Lower the heat and simmer for 30 minutes. The pork will be cooked through, and the figs and apples will be almost completely disintegrated. Stir in the remaining salt.

Mix the cornstarch with ¼ cup water until smooth. Add a few ladles of hot fig sauce to the cornstarch mixture and then stir it into the pot. Bring to a boil. Lower the heat and simmer for 3 minutes. Stir in more salt if needed and pepper to taste.

SERVES 4 TO 6

FIRE OF LIFE PORK STEW

While related to chili and gumbo, this stew has an appeal all its own. I serve it with quinoa (see page 168) or rice. The stew gets better with time; ours was left in the refrigerator for two days before we ate it.

¼ cup teff flour

1½ pounds boneless pork shoulder, cut into 1½-inch cubes

¼ cup safflower oil

1 medium onion, cut into 1-inch chunks (about 1 cup)

6 cloves garlic, smashed and peeled

3 cups tomato purée (homemade, page 208, or sterile-pack)

1½ teaspoons filé powder

3½ cups chicken stock (any of the homemade stocks, pages 203–4, or sterile-pack)

2 cups fresh okra, the smaller the better, hard ends trimmed

2 cups frozen peas or 1½ pounds fresh peas in the pod if young and tender

1 tablespoon fresh lemon juice

Kosher salt

Freshly ground black pepper

Hot sauce—Trinidadian is excellent

Spread the teff flour onto a large dinner plate. Lightly coat each piece of pork in the teff. Heat the oil in a 4- to 5-quart braising pot over medium-high heat. When the oil shimmers, arrange the pork in an even layer in the pot and brown on all sides, about 1 minute per side. Add the onion, garlic, tomato purée, filé powder, and chicken stock. Bring to a boil and reduce the heat to simmer. Cook, covered, for 1 hour. Twenty minutes before the stew is done, stir in the okra. Five minutes before the stew is done, add the peas—unless mellowing stew in the refrigerator for a day or two.

To reheat, cook, covered, over medium heat until warm enough to eat. Ten minutes after it has started cooking, add the peas.

Season the stew with the lemon juice and salt, pepper, and hot sauce to taste (be careful and add it gradually).

SERVES 4 TO 6

LAMB

I don't mean "mutton dressed up as spring lamb." There are times—usually in England—when I like mutton; but this chapter addresses lamb. The recipes run the gamut from roast leg of lamb to more unusual recipes that I have found delicious and unctuous.

LEG OF LAMB, FENNEL SEEDS, AND ORANGE

The strong flavors of the marinade are not as apparent in the lamb itself, so this subtle dish should not be served with strong-tasting vegetables like ramps or garlic that would overpower the taste of the lamb. Pungent side dishes like curry or other heavily spiced foods should also be avoided. I made the mistake; that's how I know.

This recipe needs to be started at least a day ahead to let the marinade soak in.

¼ cup fresh orange juice

2 tablespoons freshly grated orange zest

1½ tablespoons fennel seeds

1 tablespoon dried marjoram

8 cloves garlic (about 1 ounce), smashed and peeled

2 tablespoons sugar

¾ cup plus 1½ tablespoons olive oil

1 short leg of lamb, trimmed (about 5½ pounds), chops removed

1 cup white wine

Purée the orange juice, zest, fennel, marjoram, garlic, sugar, and ¾ cup olive oil in a blender until smooth. Coat the entire leg of lamb thoroughly with the marinade and put it in a plastic bag. Seal the bag and place in the refrigerator overnight (or for up to 2 days if planning well enough in advance), making sure to turn the bag every so often.

Remove the lamb from the refrigerator and bring to room temperature. Heat the oven to 500°F with a rack on the second level from the bottom.

Rub the bottom of an 18-×-13-×-2-inch roasting pan with the remaining oil.

Remove the lamb from the bag and place in the pan. Pour the marinade all over the leg. Roast for 10 minutes. Turn the lamb over and reduce the heat to 425°F. Roast another 35 minutes. Move the lamb to a platter.

Put the pan on top of the stove. Add the wine. Bring to a boil and continuously scrape the bottom of the pan with a wooden spoon. Let reduce by half. Serve in a sauceboat on the side with the lamb.

SERVES 6 TO 8

AMPLE LAMB AND MUSHROOM STEW

This is a wonderful stew for a party—even a buffet. It is a one-dish meal that could take a green salad. I make its warm richness in winter using the ingredients that I have put up at the end of summer. Readily available market ingredients can be substituted. The only thing that really would need to be made ahead is lamb stock, and chicken stock can be used instead.

½ cup olive oil

3½ pounds boneless leg of lamb, cut into 1-inch cubes

1 pound white pearl onions, peeled (see Note)

1 pound white mushrooms, trimmed and quartered (about 6 cups)

2 tablespoons ground cumin

2 cups fresh shiitake mushrooms, stemmed, cut into thin strips, and cooked briefly in a small amount of chicken stock until limp

2 cups Oyster Mushroom (*Pleurotus*) Base (page 209)

Large handful fresh oregano

Large handful fresh thyme

1 cup lamb stock or chicken stock (any of the homemade stocks, pages 203–4, or sterile-pack)

6 cloves garlic, smashed and peeled

4 cups cooked (see page 216) or drained canned navy or cannellini beans

Juice of 2 oranges

Kosher salt

In a heavy pan large enough to hold the lamb in a single layer and deep enough to hold the entire stew (I use a 12- to 13-inch-wide braising pan), heat the olive oil until shimmering. Add the lamb, stirring from time to time, until lightly browned. Add the onions and white mushrooms. When the mushrooms are slightly cooked, add the cumin. Stir well and add the cooked shiitake and the oyster mushrooms.

Wrap the herbs in a large square of cheesecloth and sink into the stew. Add the stock. Cook over medium-low heat for about 1½ hours or until the lamb is cooked but not mushy. Add the garlic along with the beans about 20 minutes before the lamb should be done.

Just before serving, add the orange juice and salt if desired.

SERVES 8 TO 10

NOTE

For easier peeling, boil the pearl onions for 1 minute, allow to cool, and then peel.

MOROCCAN LAMB STEW

A wonderful friend and co-cook for more years than either of us wishes to count is Paula Wolfert, the author—among many other books—of *Couscous and Other Good Food from Morocco*. I have never been to Morocco; but Paula has introduced me to couscous, tagines, preserved lemons, and other delights. This recipe is not her fault, and the "Preserved" Lemons are not as she would make them, but I have not been able to keep the real thing on hand. The one I make works for me. The seasonings are traditional, though not necessarily in this combination. I loved the result and hope that you will also. If you can find teff (see page 169), it is an ideal accompaniment.

Be careful when adding salt; the "Preserved" Lemons are very salty.

¼ cup safflower oil

1 medium onion, cut into ¼-inch dice (about 1½ cups)

2 pounds boneless lamb shoulder, cut into 1½-inch pieces (about 3 cups)

2 tablespoons ras el hanout

1 tablespoon sumac

1 cup chicken stock (any of the homemade stocks, pages 203–4, or sterile-pack)

1 pound zucchini, trimmed and cut into ¼-inch dice (about 4 cups)

6 to 7 cloves garlic, smashed, peeled, and roughly chopped (about ¼ cup)

3 tablespoons finely chopped cilantro (coriander) leaves

12 "Preserved" Lemon wedges (page 202)

Kosher salt

Heat the oil in a 6-quart braising pot over high heat. When the oil shimmers, reduce the heat to medium and add the onion. Cook until translucent, 3 to 4 minutes, stirring occasionally.

Toss the lamb cubes in a large bowl with the ras el hanout and sumac until coated evenly. Add the lamb to the braising pot with the onion and brown on all sides, another 3 to 4 minutes. Pour in the chicken stock and zucchini and bring to a boil, then reduce the heat to low. Cook for 40 minutes. The recipe can be made up to 2 hours ahead to this point and then reheated. Add the garlic, cilantro, and lemon wedges and cook for 5 minutes more. Season with salt to taste.

SERVES 4 TO 6

HARICOT LAMB

Another lamb stew, this time in the French tradition, rather related to a cassoulet.

14 ounces dried navy or other small white beans, rinsed (about 2 cups)

1 bay leaf

3 sprigs parsley

1 large sprig thyme

3 leaves sage

2 teaspoons kosher salt, plus more to taste

Freshly ground black pepper

1¾ pounds leg of lamb, boned and cut into 1½-inch pieces

2 tablespoons safflower oil

1 medium onion, cut into 1-inch chunks (about 1 cup)

2 cloves garlic, smashed, peeled, and crushed

2 medium potatoes (about 1 pound), peeled and cut into ½-inch chunks (about 3 cups)

½ cup tomato purée (homemade, page 208, or sterile-pack)

½ cup cornstarch (optional)

In a medium saucepan, bring enough water to cover the beans to a boil. Add the beans. Turn off the heat. Allow to sit for 30 minutes. Drain. Put the beans back into the pan. Cover with water by 4 inches. Bring to a boil. Reduce the heat and simmer until three-quarters cooked, about 20 minutes. Drain. Rinse with cold water. Set aside.

Heat the oven to 350°F with a rack in the bottom third.

Tie the bay leaf, parsley, thyme, and sage together with string or cheesecloth. Set aside.

Combine the salt with pepper to taste in a bowl. Add the lamb and toss to coat.

Warm the oil in a deep 10-inch-wide pot or Dutch oven. Add half the lamb and onion. Cook over high heat until well browned. Remove from the pan and reserve. Add the remaining lamb and onion to the pan. Cook until browned.

Stir in the reserved lamb and onion, along with the herbs, garlic, potatoes, tomato purée, beans, and 3 cups water. Cover and bake for 1 hour, until the lamb and beans are tender. Season with salt and pepper to taste.

For a thicker stew, make a slurry of cornstarch and ½ cup cold water and stir it into the lamb mixture, beating until thickened. Discard the bouquet garni before serving.

SERVES 5 OR 6

GROUND LAMB AND FLAGEOLETS

Flageolets—small pale green dried beans—are a classic with roast lamb in Bordeaux. I decided to have a little fun with the dish and think it turned out rather well. As with all dried bean dishes, this has to be started ahead by soaking the beans. If flageolets are unavailable, substitute cranberry beans. If time is of the essence, use defrosted frozen baby lima beans.

    1 cup dried flageolets (see page 214)
    2 tablespoons vegetable oil
    1 medium onion, finely diced (about 1 cup)
    3 cloves garlic, smashed, peeled, and finely chopped
    ½ pound ground lamb
    ½ cup basil leaves, cut across into ¼-inch strips
    1½ cups crushed tomatoes, fresh or sterile-pack
    Kosher salt
    Freshly ground black pepper

Soak and cook the beans according to the directions on page 216. There should be 2⅔ cups of cooked flageolets.

Heat the oil in a 14-inch sauté pan or a 12-inch braising pan over low heat. Sauté the onion and garlic until soft. Add the lamb and cook, stirring, until lightly browned. Add the basil, tomatoes, and beans and simmer for 10 minutes. Add salt and pepper to taste.

SERVES 4

CIVET OF MUTTON

To every rule there is an exception. Here is one: a recipe for mutton. It may be hard to get mutton, in which case use lamb. Classically, civet is thickened with blood, more than probably unavailable. I have compensated by making a strong-tasting dish that needs to be prepared over several days. The chicken livers compensate for the absence of blood. The stew would be relaxing to make on a skiing vacation as you don't need to stand over it the whole time and it gives intense rewards.

    One 5¼- to 5½-pound leg of mutton or lamb, boned
        and meat cut into 2-inch pieces, bones reserved,
        if available
    1 cup olive oil
    1 medium carrot, peeled and cut into ⅛-inch rounds
        (about ½ cup)
    1 small onion, cut across into ⅛-inch rounds
        (about ½ cup)
    2 medium shallots (1½ ounces), coarsely chopped
        (about ¼ cup)
    ½ stalk celery, peeled and coarsely chopped
        (scant ¼ cup)
    ⅛ cup packed parsley leaves
    2 bay leaves
    ⅛ teaspoon dried thyme
    ⅛ teaspoon ground cloves
    ⅛ teaspoon cayenne pepper
    ½ teaspoon dried rosemary
    ½ teaspoon dried juniper berries
    1 teaspoon dried sage
    1 teaspoon dried basil
    1 teaspoon quatre épices
    2 cloves garlic, smashed, peeled, and coarsely chopped
    7 cups red wine
    1 cup red wine vinegar
    2 tablespoons sugar
    2½ tablespoons kosher salt, or more to taste

3 ounces very lean bacon, sliced ⅛ inch thick and cut across into 2-inch lengths

1½ pounds small white mushrooms, about 1½-inch diameter each, trimmed

¼ cup fresh lemon juice

½ pound chicken livers, cleaned (see page 34)

½ cup cornstarch

Freshly ground black pepper

FOR AN OPTIONAL MEAT GLAZE: Put the bones in a pot and cover with water or any unsalted stock by 1 inch. Bring to a boil. Skim the broth. Reduce the heat to a very low simmer. Cook, uncovered, for 12 hours or as long as the meat marinates (see below). If necessary, add more water or stock from time to time.

FOR THE MARINADE: Put the olive oil, carrot, onion, shallots, and celery in a medium stockpot over medium-low heat. Cook for 10 minutes, until the vegetables are soft. Move them to a square of cheesecloth. Add the parsley, herbs, and spices to the cheesecloth, tie into a loose bundle, and put back into the pot. Add the garlic, wine, vinegar, sugar, and 1½ tablespoons of the salt. Bring to a boil. Reduce the heat to a good simmer and cook for 10 minutes. Transfer the marinade to a deep 11-inch-wide stockpot. Cool for 2 hours or until just slightly warm.

Add the meat to the marinade, turning the pieces to coat. Marinate, uncovered, at room temperature for 12 hours or up to 24 hours if the room is cool or cold. Remove the cheesecloth bundle and squeeze out the liquids.

FINISH THE MEAT GLAZE: Remove the bones from the stock. Strain the liquid and put it back into the pot. Bring to a boil. Cook over medium heat until reduced to 1 cup. Reserve ½ cup for use in the stew. Save the rest as a dividend for other dishes.

COOK THE MUTTON: Transfer the meat to a colander or two sieves. The oil will have risen to the top of the marinade. Use a large spoon to remove as much oil as possible and reserve.

Heat the reserved oil in a large wide pot (use two if necessary). Add the bacon and meat. Cook for 20 minutes, turning the pieces to brown on all sides. Reduce the heat and cook for 25 minutes. Add the reserved marinade and ½ cup meat glaze. Bring to a boil. Reduce the heat and simmer for 30 minutes. Cool in the refrigerator. Remove the fat that will rise to the top and solidify. Allow the stew to come to room temperature.

An hour before the final cooking of the meat, trim the mushrooms by cutting the stems flush with the caps. Halve them. Toss with the lemon juice. Set aside.

Forty-five minutes to an hour before serving, add the mushrooms to the stew. Bring to a boil. Reduce the heat and simmer.

While the stew is simmering, place half the livers and cornstarch in a blender with ¼ cup stew liquid. Purée until smooth. Repeat with the remaining livers, cornstarch, and another ¼ cup stew liquid.

After the stew has cooked for 25 minutes, stir in the liver purée. Raise the heat to a good simmer and cook, stirring constantly, until thickened. Season with the remaining 1 tablespoon salt and lots of pepper to taste.

The finished stew can be served now, kept warm over a simmer burner or a burner at lowest heat with a heat diffuser on top, or refrigerated and brought back to temperature very slowly with a heat diffuser. Serve with rice, gluten-free noodles, or steamed small new potatoes.

SERVES 10 TO 12

NIFTY NECK OF LAMB

Lamb neck is not a cut that usually springs readily to mind; but I wanted to make a deep-tasting braise/stew, and lamb neck has an ideal ratio of bone to meat to give a lovely, silky, gelatinous texture. I used half a neck, but the recipe can easily be doubled as long as a pan is used that is just large enough to hold the lamb in a single layer. Cut off any semi-attached pieces of meat and add them to the pan.

The half neck is enough to feed four as this is rich. I served it with fingerling potatoes in their skins. Rice noodles would be fine as well.

> ¼ cup olive oil
>
> 2½ pounds neck of lamb (about ½ neck), cut into 4-inch-long pieces
>
> 1 pound yellow onions, halved and thinly sliced (about 4 cups)
>
> 1 cup red wine
>
> ¼ cup fresh lemon juice
>
> Kosher salt

Heat the oil in an 8-inch saucepan until shimmering but not smoking. Add the lamb pieces and brown lightly, turning them from time to time. Add the onions and red wine. Bring to a boil and cover. Reduce the heat to simmer and cook for 30 minutes. Push the softened onions down into the liquid. Re-cover and cook for an hour. Add the lemon juice and salt to taste.

SERVES 4

HERB-SIMMERED LEG OF LAMB

European chefs have created some classic dishes pairing poached meats and flavorful sauces. There is, for example, the Italian dish *vitello tonnato*, poached veal served cold and thinly sliced in a tuna fish sauce. The French dine on *boeuf à la ficelle*, poached beef filet, sliced to show off its rosy interior and served cold with any one of a number of sauces. Such dishes are delicious and hearty enough to please a crowd of meat eaters without being too heavy.

Inspired by the classics, my leg of lamb is very good cold with a sardine sauce that is a variation on the tuna sauce made in Italy. An enriched vinaigrette can be used as an alternative, its anchovies and capers making it a tasty fish-meets-meat combination.

You can also substitute pork loin as the meat and cook it in the same way.

Remember to turn the meat in the pot so it will cook evenly. This is particularly important since the lamb will swell up and not be fully covered by the liquid at all times.

> 1 bay leaf
>
> 4 medium cloves garlic, unpeeled
>
> 2 teaspoons dried rosemary
>
> One 2¾-pound boneless leg of lamb, rolled and tied
>
> Sardine Sauce (page 196) or Enriched Vinaigrette (page 195)

In a 10½-inch-wide braising pan or stockpot, bring 4 quarts water to a boil with the bay leaf, garlic, and rosemary. Add the lamb and return to a boil. Lower the heat and simmer for 1½ hours, turning the lamb every 20 minutes.

Remove the pot from the stove and allow the meat to cool in the liquid. Remove the meat from the liquid and slice across into ¼-inch-thick slices; there should be 25 to 30 slices.

Spread a cup of sardine sauce on a medium platter or in a baking dish. Place a layer of lamb slices on top of the sauce and then spread the slices with more sauce. Continue until all of the sauce and meat have been used. Cover with plastic wrap and refrigerate for 1 hour or up to 3 days. If you are using the enriched vinaigrette instead, simply drizzle it over the sliced meat just before serving.

SERVES 10

OTHER MEATS

These are the pieces that most people seem to eat in restaurants. When I can get good pieces, I relish them at home. I don't insist that they be tried; but they are worth the eating. Chicken livers are covered on pages 33–34 of "Hors d'Oeuvre & First Courses."

SAUTÉED CALVES' LIVER WITH BACON

Even I don't eat pork liver, finding the taste too strong. Various dogs that I have had over the years loved it. Kosher calves' liver is finer and lighter in taste than other kinds. It's worth asking if it is available. All liver is good against anemia.

If the liver has a membrane around it, pull it off. Hope that your butcher has removed any large veins. If not, they will need to be cut out.

4 thick strips bacon (about 4 ounces)

1 large onion, finely chopped (about 1 cup)

1 tablespoon safflower oil

1 pound calves' liver sliced ½ inch thick, outer membrane removed, cut into 4 pieces

Freshly ground black pepper

Cook the bacon over medium-high heat in a 10-inch skillet until crisp, 3 to 4 minutes. Put on a plate. Add the onion to the hot pan and cook until soft and translucent, 4 to 5 minutes. Move the onion to another plate. Pour the safflower oil into the pan. Place two pieces of liver in the pan at a time. Cook just until brown, about 30 seconds a side for rare liver. Move to a serving platter. Repeat with the remaining pieces. Place the bacon and onion on top of the cooked liver. Add pepper to taste. Serve immediately.

SERVES 2

SWEETBREADS WITH CAPER AND LEMON SAUCE

It is too bad that sweetbreads are usually served and eaten only in restaurants. They are easy and quick to make, and actually most people love them.

Try to avoid capers packed in vinegar. A good Italian store or online market should be able to supply salt-packed capers. Oddly enough, small ones are better than big ones.

Basic teff (see page 169) makes a good accompaniment, or serve Simple Spring Vegetables (page 146) as I did.

2 cups chicken stock (any of the homemade stocks, pages 203–4, or sterile-pack)

2 tablespoons capers in salt (do not rinse them)

1 tablespoon fresh lemon juice

½ cup rice bran

1½ pounds sweetbreads, cleaned (see sidebar, opposite) and cut into approximately 4-inch pieces

Safflower oil

In a small saucepan over medium-low heat, reduce the chicken stock to 1 cup. Stir in the capers and lemon juice. Set aside.

Spread the rice bran on a large dinner plate. Individually turn the sweetbread pieces until well coated.

Pour oil ¼ inch deep into a 10- to 12-inch skillet over high heat. When the oil shimmers, gently place the sweetbread pieces in an even layer in the pan. As soon as they brown (they will brown quickly) turn them over and cook on the other side until browned. Put on a platter and pour the caper sauce over the top.

SERVES 4

VARIATION

Calves' Brains with Caper and Lemon Sauce

To cook calves' brains, make sure to trim away the brain stem (it is a bright white tube extending downward from the brain). Also, separate the two lobes (halves) of the brain by trimming away the white connective tissue that joins them.

Two brains should weigh just under 1 pound, so each lobe is roughly 4 ounces. Dredge the cleaned lobes in rice bran and continue as directed, cooking the pieces for 5 minutes on one side and 4 to 5 minutes more on the other side.

SERVES 4

- -

SWEETBREADS

Sweetbreads are the set of glands of veal (technically, they are also found in young beef, lamb, and pork, but veal sweetbreads are by far the most delicious and most readily available). One of these elongated glands, the thymus gland, is found right by the throat; the other, the pancreas gland—which is larger, round, and plump—is found near the heart. They can be purchased fresh at your local butcher if you call in advance, or bought frozen from other vendors. The set of glands usually weighs about 1¼ pounds.

Most people don't make these at home. It's too bad, because they are delicious and, once cleaned, cook quickly.

1 pair sweetbreads (1¼ pounds)

CLEANING

To clean, first manually remove all visible fat, blood vessels, and veins. The fat will appear as little hard white pebbles. The blood vessels are bright red, and the veins are rubbery and white. This can all be trimmed away with a knife, but I find it more effective (and less wasteful) to pull all the undesirable pieces out of the glands by hand. The glands are encased in a thin, translucent membrane that needs to be removed before cooking. Make an incision with a sharp knife in the center of the smoother side of the gland and peel away the membrane. It takes some coaxing, but the membrane can be separated from the pink flesh underneath. Do not be alarmed if the glands start to break apart. The gland will separate into different pieces, large and small. Larger portions can be panfried as is or trimmed into more manageable pieces while little nuggets are ideal for deep-frying.

- -

APPLE-CIDER-RICH BOILED TONGUE DINNER

This requires that the family not be squeamish eaters. I start with a raw tongue, but it's okay to buy a cooked one.

> **12 medium new potatoes**
>
> **15 white boiling onions (each 1 to 1½ inches in diameter), peeled**
>
> **1½ cups dark beer**
>
> **5 cups apple cider**
>
> **1 cup apple cider vinegar**
>
> **½ teaspoon ground cloves**
>
> **2 teaspoons sugar**
>
> **1 tablespoon kosher salt**
>
> **6 small carrots, peeled, cut in half lengthwise, and then across into 2-inch pieces**
>
> **1 large head garlic (about 20 cloves), smashed and peeled**
>
> **One 1½-pound piece cooked beef tongue, skin and fibers removed**
>
> **1 medium head green cabbage, cut into 6 wedges through the core**

Place the potatoes, onions, beer, cider, vinegar, cloves, sugar, and salt in a large wide pot over high heat. Cover. Bring to a boil. Lower the heat and cook, covered, at a moderate boil for 10 minutes.

Add the carrots, garlic, and tongue, pushing the vegetables away as much as possible to allow the tongue to nestle in the liquid. Cover. Return to a boil. Lower the heat and cook, covered, at a moderate boil for 5 minutes.

Lay the cabbage wedges on top of the other ingredients. Cover. Return to a boil. Lower the heat and cook, covered, at a moderate boil for 20 minutes or until the cabbage is tender.

Serve slices of tongue, along with a variety of the vegetables, in a large rimmed bowl with a bit of the broth. (The tongue can also be presented on a large platter with the vegetables. The broth can be served on the side.)

SERVES 6

VEAL TONGUE

The rich but not domineering flavors of the Marsala and mushrooms make this an elegant dish. It can be multiplied to serve as many as desired.

> 1 to 1¼ pounds veal tongue
> ½ cup Marsala
> 1 ounce dried porcini
> Kosher salt
> Freshly ground black pepper

In an 8-inch saucepan, bring enough water to a boil to cover the tongue. Add the tongue. Reduce the heat to a low boil and cook for 1 hour and 15 minutes.

While the tongue is cooking, put the dried mushrooms and Marsala in a 2-cup glass measure. Microwave for 1 minute. Using a skimmer or slotted spoon, lift out the mushrooms. Strain the liquid through cheesecloth or a fine sieve. Put the mushrooms back in the liquid and set aside.

Put the tongue on a plate and reserve the liquid.

Allow the tongue to cool slightly. Hold it with a cloth. Pull off the thick skin, using a sharp knife if needed to loosen the skin where it sticks. Cut off the root ends. Save them for the dog, who will be ecstatic.

Add enough of the reserved cooking liquid to the mushroom mixture to cover. Cook in a microwave oven or small pan on the stovetop for a minute. Stir and cook for a minute more.

Thinly slice the tongue crosswise and put in a small saucepan with the mushroom mixture. If needed, add enough of the reserved cooking liquid to cover. Bring to a low boil and simmer for 20 minutes. Add salt and pepper to taste. Serve with boiled rice and a side salad to one vigorous or two more fastidious eaters.

MAKES 1½ CUPS

CLEANING KIDNEYS

I think part of the reason people don't try to eat kidneys at home is that they don't know how to clean and cook them. Here are a few notes to help those adventurous home cooks.

SMALL KIDNEYS

Cleaning the kidneys is easy with sharp kitchen scissors. Cut the kidneys in half lengthwise along the side with the white dot. There will be a strip of white running down the length of each half. Holding the white strip with one hand and using the scissors with the other, ease the red meat away from the white strip until only the tips of the white strips attach to the meat. Snip off each attachment. It all sounds more complicated than it is. Once mastered, it will go quickly.

LARGE KIDNEYS

The large ones that I found required a different manner of cleaning than small kidneys. Grab the kidneys one by one by the white part that protrudes. Carefully slide the tips of sharp kitchen scissors down one side of the white veins, gently cutting the meat loose. When one side is complete, rotate the kidney to do the same thing on another side. Keep doing this until the veins are attached to the meat at the very bottom. Snip the veins loose. Set the kidneys aside—in my case, on a high counter to thwart the dog, who seems enchanted by the smell.

KIDNEYS AND KUMQUATS

I have a dear friend, Paula Frosch, who, upon hearing that I was having trouble getting kidneys to test recipes with, provided me a supply of kidneys through a friend who is a farmer-cum-butcher in Massachusetts. They turned out to be pork kidneys, which I had never cooked. The flavor and texture are much the same as those of lamb kidneys, but different from veal kidneys.

The kidneys varied greatly in size, from small ones that obviously came from suckling pigs to larger ones that weighed a little more than an ounce each. I developed this recipe and the two recipes that follow using these large pork kidneys, but then adapted them all for lamb kidneys, which are easier to get.

I found that the easiest way to clean them was to quarter them lengthwise and then to proceed with scissors as in the general instructions opposite.

The idea of using kumquats did not leap into my mind full blown. Rather, I was walking through the market, idly wondering what to buy and use. I saw the kumquats and thought that their astringent acidity would be good with the kidneys, as well as colorful. Kidneys do not cook to a wonderful color. Even after cooking, the dish wasn't beautiful; the kumquats darkened as they cooked and softened. I had some pomegranates and sprinkled the seeds on top. That did the trick, both visually and by adding a lovely fresh pop.

¼ cup safflower oil

About 9½ ounces lamb kidneys, cleaned and cut into 8 pieces, about 4 pieces per kidney

¼ pound whole kumquats (about 1 cup), plus a few extra for garnish

½ cup hard cider or regular cider

2 tablespoons potato starch

Kosher salt

Freshly ground black pepper

2 pomegranates, seeded

Heat the oil over high heat in a 10-inch sauté pan, until it shimmers. Add the kidney pieces and cook, stirring, for 1 minute. Turn the pieces over and cook for 30 seconds. Stir in the kumquats and cook for 40 seconds. Add the cider and bring to a boil.

Stir the potato starch into ¼ cup water. Stir some of the cooking liquid from the pan into the potato starch mixture. Add the mixture to the pan. Turn off the heat and let cook by retained heat until thickened. Add salt and pepper to taste. Sprinkle each portion with some of the pomegranate seeds. Put an uncooked kumquat in the center of each portion. Serve with rice or another starch.

SERVES 4 TO 6

LAMB KIDNEYS

I know, yuck. Even my fabulous editor, Ann Bramson, would not eat them, let alone the two Chilean women who work with me. I made them, coerced the people, and surprise, a miracle: they ate them eagerly after a gingerly first taste. Three kidneys make a serving; but if tentative, serve one or half of one as a first course. They would be attractive on a bed of watercress.

The rice bran used for the coating is the only exotic ingredient here, but it is well worth having on hand as it is one of the best and only cleaners of arteries and blood veins. When I first tried it as a health supplement, I hated it; but now that I have found its proper role in life, I will try it often instead of flour or bread crumbs for coating. It gives a lovely crunch.

The mayonnaise-mustard combination makes enough for four kidneys if feeling brave.

2 plump lamb kidneys (about ¼ pound each), halved and cleaned (see page 140)

⅓ cup mayonnaise (homemade, page 190, or store-bought)

¼ cup Dijon mustard

2 tablespoons fresh lemon juice

¼ cup rice bran

2 tablespoons olive oil

Place the cleaned kidney halves to one side. Whisk together the mayonnaise, mustard, and lemon juice. Put a layer of the rice bran in a flat soup bowl. Turn the kidney halves in the marinade until completely coated. Gently pick the halves up one by one and place on the rice bran. Allow to sit a few minutes. Gently turn them over. The point is to get a nice coating.

Heat the olive oil in a sauté pan large enough to hold the kidney halves in one layer. Heat the oil over high heat, then turn the heat down to medium. Gently lay the pieces of kidney in the hot oil and cook for 3 minutes. With a pancake spatula, turn them over and cook for 3 minutes more. Eat immediately.

SERVES 1 OR 2

LAMB KIDNEY DELIGHT

This title may seem like an oxymoron; but it describes this dish. It is just important to know that your guests don't have a repugnance to kidneys. It makes a good amount of luscious sauce, but I don't thicken it. I prefer to offer spoons of polenta, quinoa, or grits to give guests tastes of the delicious sauce.

The only real work is cleaning the kidneys. The rest goes very quickly.

> ¼ pound sliced bacon, sliced across in ¼-inch strips
>
> 2 tablespoons olive oil
>
> 2 pounds mild onions, cut into quarters and thinly sliced across
>
> 2 pounds lamb kidneys, cleaned (see page 140)
>
> 1 pound oyster mushrooms or other mild firm mushrooms, cut lengthwise into ½-inch-wide slices
>
> ½ cup apple cider
>
> 1 tablespoon horseradish
>
> Kosher salt
>
> Freshly ground black pepper

Put the bacon slices in a heavy pan with a tablespoon of the olive oil. Sauté over medium heat until the bacon begins to give off its fat. Add the onions and kidneys. When the onions have softened, move to a separate dish.

Add the mushrooms to the same pan and sauté for about 3 minutes. Pour on the apple cider and the horseradish and stir for about 3 minutes. Add back the kidney mixture and stir until warm. Add salt and pepper to taste and serve.

SERVES 4 AS A MAIN COURSE, 6 AS A FIRST COURSE

SEASONAL VEAL KIDNEYS

These are seasonal not only because they are so good in the fall but also because this recipe adds lots of flavor. Like much of the world today, meat seems to arrive Cryovac-ed. Kidneys usually come two to a package, with each weighing about 1¼ pounds. In this recipe they lie in a lovely marinade for about an hour, not to tenderize them—they are already tender—but to add rich flavor. The marinade makes about ⅔ cup sauce. Serve with rice or with Olive Oil Mashed Potatoes (page 165).

> 5 garlic cloves, smashed and peeled
>
> 2 ounces ginger, peeled and thinly sliced
>
> ¼ cup gluten-free soy sauce
>
> 5 drops toasted sesame oil
>
> ¼ cup mirin
>
> 2 veal kidneys (one 2½-pound package), cleaned (see page 140) and halved

Put all the ingredients except the kidneys in a blender and purée. Pour into a flat dish long enough to hold the flat kidney pieces. Put the four pieces of kidney in the dish with the marinade. Allow to sit for about 2 hours, turning from time to time.

Heat the oven to 500°F. Put the kidney pieces and marinade in a roasting pan. Cook for 25 minutes. Five minutes before the end of the cooking time, pour in 1 cup water, scraping the bottom of the pan.

Remove from the oven and thinly slice on the diagonal.

SERVES 8

VEGETABLE MAIN COURSES

This chapter includes only main-course vegetable dishes. The next chapter will cover both recipes for side dishes made from vegetables that we all enjoy and those starches that I use instead of wheat-based dishes.

BRUNCH BEAUTY

There are hundreds of recipes based on poached eggs. This recipe is inspired by Eggs Florentine (page 18), a classic in which the eggs nestle in a bed of creamed spinach. It has been made even more luscious by replacing the original bécha-mel sauce with Roe Sauce. More detailed instructions on egg poaching can be found on page 19. SEE COLOR PLATE 13

> 2 pounds fresh spinach or 1½ packages (15 ounces total) frozen chopped spinach
>
> 4 eggs
>
> ½ teaspoon olive oil
>
> ½ cup Roe Sauce (page 191)

If using fresh spinach, stem, wash well, and cook in a heavy pan until limp. Drain thoroughly in a sieve, pressing to remove as much water as possible. Pulse in a food processor until coarsely chopped and strain again. If using frozen spin-ach, defrost in a sieve under hot running water. Press with the back of a spoon to remove as much water as possible.

Bring 2 inches of water to a boil in a 9-inch saucepan. Break each egg into a demitasse cup with a rounded bot-tom. Smoothly pour the eggs into the water and poach for 2 to 3 minutes, until as firm as desired. Using a slotted spoon, remove each to a bowl of warm water.

Grease the inside of a 9-inch pie plate or quiche dish with the oil.

Heat the broiler with a rack at the highest level of the oven. Make a smooth layer of the spinach in the oiled pan. With the back of a kitchen spoon, make four depressions that do not touch and that are about 1 inch from the edge of the pan. Drain the eggs. Place one in each depression. Divide the sauce to cover the eggs. Do not let sauce touch the sides of the pan. Place the pan on a cookie sheet and broil for 4 minutes.

SERVES 4

SIMPLE SPRING VEGETABLES WITH PASTA

This vegetarian dish can be served as a main course, as a pasta course, or, without pasta, as a side dish.

I was very lucky to find tiny sugar snaps that didn't need stringing, but most will. SEE COLOR PLATE 9

> ¾ pound green beans, tipped and tailed
>
> ½ cup olive oil
>
> 1 medium onion, cut into ¼-inch dice
>
> ½ pound cremini mushrooms, trimmed and sliced across ¼ inch thick
>
> ¼ cup dried morel mushroom (porcini also work well)
>
> ½ pound sugar snap peas, trimmed and strings removed
>
> Kosher salt
>
> Freshly ground black pepper
>
> 1 pound gluten-free spaghettini, capellini, or other thin pasta (see page 39), cooked

Bring 3 quarts water to a boil in a large saucepan. Add the beans. Cook until tender enough to be split with a fork, 8 to 10 minutes (cooking time will vary depending on the age of the beans). Drain. Set aside.

Pour the oil into a 10- to 12-inch skillet over medium heat. Add the onion. Cook until translucent, about 5 minutes. Stir in the fresh mushrooms and cook for 2 to 3 minutes more. Set aside.

Place the dried mushrooms in a 2-cup glass measure with ½ cup water. Cover tightly with plastic wrap and microwave on high for 3 minutes. Drain. With scissors, cut the dried mushrooms into ¼-inch pieces. Add with the snap peas to the onion-mushroom mixture and cook over medium heat for 3 to 4 minutes, stirring occasionally. When the snap peas are almost cooked through, add the cooked string beans. Season to taste with salt and pepper. Toss with the pasta.

SERVES 4 AS A MAIN COURSE, 6 AS A PASTA COURSE

VEGETABLE STEW

The thickener in this superb stew is okra, the vegetable kingdom's version of gelatin. As it cooks, it releases a viscous substance that binds together disparate ingredients. It is the keystone of gumbo (whose name stems from the Bantu word for okra), where a hodgepodge of ingredients hangs together thanks to okra.

Okra works especially well in this vegetables-only stew, which evokes the Caribbean more than Cajun country in its seasoning.

To season the vegetable stew, add the lime juice before adjusting the seasoning and adding more salt. Because the stew is so thick, with barely any liquid, the rice should be cooked separately and added at the end. The rice also makes the whole dish taste less spicy, but those with fragile taste buds can reduce the amount of hot pepper.

2 tablespoons safflower oil

1 large yellow onion, cut into ¼-inch dice

3 medium cloves garlic, smashed, peeled, and coarsely chopped

2 medium bunches chard (about 1¾ pounds), leaves removed and cut across into ¼-inch strips, stems cut across into ¼-inch slices

1 bay leaf

Large pinch ground allspice

2 medium dried hot red peppers, crumbled

1 medium butternut squash, peeled, seeded, and cut into 1-inch cubes (about 4 cups)

2 medium sweet potatoes, peeled and cut into 1-inch cubes (about 3 cups)

1 pound fresh okra, trimmed and cut across into ¼-inch rounds

2 tablespoons plus ½ teaspoon fresh lime juice, or to taste

1 tablespoon kosher salt, or to taste

4½ cups cooked white rice

In a medium stockpot, heat the oil over medium-low heat. Stir in the onion and cook, stirring occasionally, for 5 minutes. Stir in the garlic and cook, stirring occasionally, for 3 minutes or until the onion and garlic are translucent.

Stir in the chard stems and cook, stirring occasionally, for 3 minutes. Add 3 cups water, the bay leaf, allspice, and hot peppers. Cover and bring to a boil.

Stir in the squash and sweet potatoes. Cover and return to a boil. Lower the heat and simmer, covered, for 10 minutes.

Add the chard greens and the okra. Cover and return to a boil, pushing the greens and okra down into the liquid once in a while to aid the wilting.

Lower the heat slightly, cover the pot, and boil gently, stirring occasionally, for 10 minutes or until the chard and okra are cooked through. There will be very little liquid left at the end, so be careful not to let it burn. Season with lime juice and salt. Serve over the rice.

SERVES 6

CHICKPEA STEW WITH POACHED EGGS

Increasingly, I seem to have friends who are vegetarians. This robust dish is beautiful and a treat. For those who like spicier food, some harissa stirred into the vegetable stew before the eggs are added gives a good jolt. Vegans can omit the eggs.

> 2 bunches spinach, stemmed and coarsely chopped (about 4 cups)
>
> 2 cups grape or cherry tomatoes
>
> 1 cup whole roasted almonds
>
> 1 bunch scallions, trimmed, cut across into ¼-inch pieces including some of the greens (about 1 cup)
>
> Kosher salt
>
> 2 cups gluten-free dried penne pasta
>
> 1 bunch mint (about 1 ounce), stemmed and coarsely chopped (about ½ cup)
>
> 1½ tablespoons dried oregano
>
> ½ cup olive oil
>
> Freshly ground black pepper
>
> One 19-ounce can chickpeas (garbanzo beans), drained and rinsed, or 2½ cups cooked chickpeas (see page 221)
>
> 6 eggs

Pour 2 cups water into a 4- to 5-quart saucepan over medium heat. When the water begins to steam, drop in the spinach. Cook until the spinach is dark green and wilted, about 2 minutes. Add the tomatoes, almonds, and scallions. Simmer for 5 minutes.

Bring 3 quarts water and 2 tablespoons salt to a boil in a large saucepan over high heat. Drop the pasta into the pot and cook for 7 minutes. While the pasta is cooking, add the mint, oregano, oil, 1 tablespoon salt, and pepper to taste to the vegetables, along with the chickpeas. Drain the pasta and add to the vegetables. Stir well and cook for a minute. (The dish can be made ahead until this point. To finish, put the stew in a 14-inch skillet and return to a simmer. Proceed as follows.)

Put the stew into a 14-inch skillet. Make sure the tomatoes and almonds are distributed evenly throughout the pan. Using the bottom of a soup ladle, make 6 deep indentations along the edges of the stew. Carefully crack an egg into each of the indents. Cover the skillet and cook for 3 to 4 minutes, until the whites have set but the yolks are still runny.

SERVES 4 TO 6

TORTILLA ESPAÑOLA

When I first ate the flat, browned omelets, I was confused. In Spain they are called *tortillas* and are not like the Central American flatbreads. They are good at breakfast, at lunch, or as a first course at dinner. A good tomato sauce (see page 193) goes well.

1 tablespoon plus ½ teaspoon olive oil

½ bunch spinach (3 ounces), stemmed (about 2 cups)

1 small potato (Yukon Gold or new potato works nicely), peeled and sliced ⅛ inch thick on a box grater or mandoline (about 1 cup)

6 eggs

¼ cup chopped chives (about ½ bunch)

Kosher salt

Freshly ground black pepper

Preheat the oven to 375°F with a rack in the middle. Heat 1½ teaspoons of the oil in an 8-inch nonstick ovenproof sauté pan over medium heat. Add the spinach and cook until the leaves wilt and turn dark green, about a minute. Move the spinach to a plate.

Add the remaining 2 teaspoons oil to the pan and arrange the potato slices in an even layer. Cook until the edges begin to brown, 2 to 3 minutes. Flip the potatoes over and cook for 2 minutes more, until almost fully cooked. Whisk the eggs together in a medium bowl until well combined. Spread the cooked spinach evenly on top of the potatoes. Pour the eggs over the vegetables. Cook until the edges of the egg mixture have turned opaque and begun to brown, about 5 minutes. Sprinkle the chives over the eggs and season with salt and pepper to taste. Transfer the pan to the oven and bake for 15 minutes.

Slide the tortilla out of the pan, cut into wedges, and serve. It can also be inverted onto a plate, cut, and served. The golden brown potatoes look just as inviting as the bright green spinach. The tortilla can be eaten warm or at room temperature.

SERVES 3 OR 4 AS A MAIN COURSE, 6 AS A FIRST COURSE

BLACK BEAN FEIJOADA OVER SPICY RICE

Feijoada is a Brazilian dish that is usually rich with every part of the pig, including the ears. This is a vegan version—still very good.

BEANS

2 cups dried black beans

1 large onion, chopped

3 cloves garlic, smashed, peeled, and minced

1 tablespoon safflower oil

6 cups Vegetable Broth (page 206) or water

1 bay leaf

¼ teaspoon freshly ground black pepper

2 oranges, whole or halved

Kosher salt

2 stalks celery, peeled and chopped

RICE

1 onion, chopped

3 cloves garlic, smashed, peeled, and minced

3 tablespoons olive oil

2 tomatoes, peeled and coarsely chopped

2½ cups cooked brown rice

SAUCE

Juice of 1 lemon

2 tomatoes, peeled

1 small onion, quartered

2 cloves garlic

1 teaspoon chili sauce

1 fresh hot green chili, stemmed (optional)

¼ cup wine or cider vinegar

Kosher salt

COOK THE BEANS: Soak the beans in stock or water overnight or at least for several hours.

In a large flameproof bean pot or Dutch oven, sauté the onion and garlic in the oil until the onion is tender. Add the drained beans, broth, bay leaf, and pepper.

Bring the beans to a boil, add the oranges, salt to taste, and the celery, and simmer, covered, for 2 to 3 hours. After the first hour, remove the lid and simmer uncovered.

When the beans are tender, remove about one-third of them and mash. Return the beans to the pot and continue cooking until the mashed beans thicken the mixture. Set aside.

PREPARE THE RICE: Sauté the onion and garlic in the olive oil over medium heat until the onion is tender and golden, about 15 minutes. Add the tomatoes and simmer for a few minutes, then stir in the cooked rice and mix well. Keep warm over low heat until ready to serve (unless you make it far in advance—then just heat over medium heat shortly before serving).

MAKE THE SAUCE: When ready to serve, put all the sauce ingredients, including salt to taste, in a blender and liquefy. Stir into the feijoada and serve over the rice.

SERVES 6 TO 8

SIDES

I divide my side dishes into two groupings. I can make a meal out of an assortment of my favorite vegetables, especially when my garden in Vermont is burgeoning. In any case, many main courses such as roasts require a vegetable-based side dish. Then come what I call "meal builders"—these feature starches such as potatoes, quinoa, teff, and polenta.

VEGETABLES

Unless the main course is a pasta dish loaded with vegetables or a stew, it will require an accompanying vegetable dish, with or without a permissible starch.

PEAS WITH CHILIES AND TOMATOES

This side dish is not spicy but smoky. If a spicier flavor is desired, Tabasco or finely chopped chili peppers added when cooking or another chili pepper sauce added at the end can suit your palate. Serve hot, warm, or cool.

> **2 pequín or bird chilies**
>
> **3 ancho chilies**
>
> **1 medium onion, finely chopped (about 1½ cups)**
>
> **1 tablespoon canola oil**
>
> **3½ pounds peas in the pod, shelled (about 4 cups)**
>
> **1¼ cups sterile-packed diced tomatoes, passed through the finest disc of a food mill**
>
> **Kosher salt**
>
> **Freshly ground black pepper**

Bring 1 quart water to a boil. Pour the boiling water over the dried chilies in a medium bowl. Cover and soak for 1½ hours. Remove the seeds and stem ends from the chilies. Purée the chilies very well in a blender. In a large, nonreactive pot, soften the onion in the oil over medium heat, about 4 minutes. Stir in the peas and cook for 2 minutes. Add the chili purée and the tomato purée. Reduce the heat to low; cook for 20 minutes or until the peas are soft. Remove from the heat and add salt and pepper to taste.

MAKES 4 CUPS

PEAS WITH MINT

Sugar is optional in this classic recipe, depending on how sweet and fresh the peas are.

> **¼ cup olive oil**
>
> **1½ pounds peas in the pod, shelled, or 2 cups frozen**
>
> **¼ cup mint leaves, cut across into thin strips**
>
> **½ head Boston lettuce, cut into ¼-inch strips (about 1½ cups)**
>
> **¼ teaspoon kosher salt**
>
> **½ teaspoon sugar (optional)**

Heat the oil in a small pan over high heat. Add the peas and cook for 2 minutes. Cover and reduce the heat to medium. Cook for 3 minutes or until the peas are tender. Stir in the mint. Cook for 2 minutes longer. Add the lettuce. Cook until the lettuce has wilted. Remove from the heat and add the salt and, if necessary, the sugar.

MAKES 2 CUPS

SAUTÉED ZUCCHINI WITH DILL

Quick and flavorful, this can be made with yellow summer squash in the fall.

> **¼ cup plus 1 tablespoon olive oil**
>
> **2 pounds young zucchini, cut into ¼-inch-thick rounds**
>
> **½ cup chopped dill**
>
> **Juice of 1 lemon**
>
> **Kosher salt**

Heat the oil in a 12-inch sauté pan. Add the zucchini, dill, and lemon juice. Cook over medium heat, stirring, until the zucchini is cooked, but still slightly crisp. Add salt to taste.

SERVES 6 TO 8

PISELLI ALLA ROMANA

As starches, peas love fat. An excellent example is the Italian preparation Piselli alla Romana, using olive oil and ham. Romans use prosciutto. I prefer the Spanish serrano as it is less likely to dry out and is less salty. This dish was given to me by Giuseppe, the attentive owner of New York's excellent Sistina restaurant. In the spring I have been known to make a whole meal of these peas.

3 large shallots, minced

3 tablespoons extra-virgin olive oil, plus more for drizzling

3½ pounds peas in the pod, shelled (about 4 cups)

2 slices prosciutto or serrano ham, cut into thin strips, then crosswise into small squares

6 cups romaine lettuce, ribs removed, shredded into thin strips

½ teaspoon kosher salt

Freshly ground black pepper

Slowly cook the shallots in the olive oil in a 12-inch skillet over very low heat until wilted, 3 to 4 minutes. Increase the heat to low. Add the peas. Cook for 15 minutes, stirring a few times. Add the ham and lettuce. Cook for 10 minutes more. Season with the salt and pepper to taste. Drizzle with olive oil.

MAKES 4 CUPS

RHUBARB WITH ASPARAGUS AND MUSHROOMS

Rhubarb completes a spring trio as a vegetable rather than a fruit when cooked with asparagus and mushrooms. I spread this on top of grilled Firm Polenta (page 171) as a first course or as a side dish with roasted chicken or fish.

And to those who think of rhubarb as a stringy, hard-to-eat vegetable, here's a tip: slice the stalks diagonally and thinly across.

2 tablespoons safflower oil

1 tablespoon toasted sesame oil

1 pound asparagus, woody stems snapped off, remaining portion peeled and cut across into 1½-inch pieces

⅓ pound oyster mushrooms (*Pleurotus*), trimmed and cut lengthwise through the stem into 2 pieces for small clusters or 3 pieces for large

4 medium stalks rhubarb, trimmed and cut diagonally into ¼-inch pieces (about 2 cups)

½ teaspoon kosher salt

½ teaspoon sugar

Lots of freshly ground black pepper

In a large skillet, heat the safflower and sesame oils over high heat until shimmering. Stir in the asparagus and mushrooms. Cook, stirring, for 2 minutes. The bottom of the pan will begin to brown.

Stir in the rhubarb. It will create enough moisture for the food not to stick or burn. Cook, stirring, for 3 minutes more. Remove from the heat and stir in the salt, sugar, and pepper. Let sit for 5 minutes before serving.

SERVES 4

LIGHT AND LOVELY BOK CHOY

Only the bok choy here is Chinese. This is cooked simply and is a perfect side dish with chicken, veal, or fish. It is amazing how much flavor the bok choy has without being gussied up with Asian seasonings.

2 tablespoons safflower oil

8 pieces baby bok choy (a little over 1 pound)

6 cloves garlic, smashed and peeled

1 cup Extra-Rich Chicken Stock (page 204) or Fake Chicken Stock (page 204)

Pick a saucepan just large enough to hold the bok choy in a single layer. Heat the oil until shimmering. Using tongs, lay in the bok choy and allow it to sizzle for about 2 minutes. Turn it over and turn down the heat to simmer. Toss in the garlic cloves and turn from time to time. Cook for 4 minutes. Turn the bok choy over and cook for 4 minutes more. Turn the heat to high and pour in the chicken stock. Bring to a boil. Lower the heat and cook at a slow boil for 5 minutes or until the thick part of the bok choy is pierced easily with a knife. No seasonings needed. Serve with a little of the cooking juice over each piece.

SERVES 4

MAGICAL GREEN TOMATOES

The triumphs of tomatoes are usually tenderness and perfume. Mostly they are bright red, although there are now heirloom varieties that are green when ripe, striped, red-brown, and various shades of yellow—to name only a few. True green ones are usually eaten raw unless they are fried coated in cornmeal as in the American South. This recipe breaks all the rules, which seems to be a specialty of mine. The assuredly unripe tomatoes are cooked into a savory side vegetable. This is definitely not a salad; it is a warm to hot side dish. I invented it due to a cold snap and inundation of tomatoes that would go bad rather than ripening. I decided to balance the acid of the green tomatoes with well-cooked onions, which achieves a rich sweetness.

⅓ cup olive oil

1¼ pounds small white onions about 1 inch in diameter, cut into thin wedges—cippoline will do nicely (about 3 cups)

4 pounds unripe green tomatoes, cored and cut into wedges about 1 inch wide

¼ cup basil leaves, cut across into thin strips

Kosher salt

Freshly ground black pepper

Choose a saucepan large enough to hold the tomatoes and still leave room for stirring. Add the olive oil to the pan and stir in the onions. Cook, stirring from time to time until the onions are fairly brown—about 15 minutes.

Add the tomatoes and cook, stirring, over low heat until liquid begins to ooze out—about 15 minutes. Turn the heat up to medium and cook, stirring, for 15 minutes more. Stir in the basil. Cooking can stop here. When ready to serve, bring the tomatoes back to medium heat and add salt and pepper to taste.

SERVES 4 TO 6 AS A SIDE DISH, 8 AS A PASTA SAUCE

ROASTED CHERRY TOMATOES WITH ORANGE AND CARDAMOM

An unusual set of seasonings, but the tomatoes seem to enjoy them. I do. SEE COLOR PLATE 14

> 2 pints stemmed cherry tomatoes (ample 4 cups)
>
> 1½ tablespoons olive oil
>
> ¼ teaspoon kosher salt, or to taste
>
> 5 strips orange zest, each ¼ inch wide and 3 inches long
>
> 5 cloves garlic, smashed, peeled, and each cut lengthwise into 4 pieces
>
> 10 cardamom pods, hit with the flat of a knife to liberate about 2 teaspoons seeds

Heat the oven to 500°F with a rack in the center.

Put the tomatoes into a shallow 9-×-13-inch roasting pan. Add the olive oil and roll the tomatoes in it until thoroughly coated. Sprinkle with the salt. Roast for 10 minutes. Shake the pan to turn the tomatoes around. Add the orange zest, garlic, and cardamom pods and seeds around the tomatoes so that they are resting on the pan. Roast for 15 minutes.

SERVES 4 TO 6

BURNISHED ENDIVE

I am very happy with this dish, with its complex, rich, meltingly deep taste. It can be a first course, allowing two or three per person, or it can be served as part of a main course. I originally devised it to go with a simple fish and polenta (see page 170) with the sauce from the endive moistening the whole. For that occasion, I used a very gelatinized, firmly set fish stock (see page 205). However, any gelatin-rich stock can be used.

Of course one can make a smaller number of endives. I did six the first time; but they keep well and are delicious. For this number of endives a very large sauté pan or braising pan (about 14 inches wide) is needed. Most large sauté pans do not come with lids, and the endive must be cooked covered. I use a cookie sheet.

If some of the outer endive leaves flop loose during the browning, don't worry, the dish will be fine. I find that tongs are necessary for turning the endives.

> 1 cup olive oil
>
> 14 medium heads Belgian endive (about 3¾ pounds), root end trimmed just to clean
>
> 2 cups Extra-Rich Chicken Stock (page 204)
>
> Kosher salt
>
> Freshly ground black pepper

Heat the olive oil in a large sauté pan or braising pan until shimmering, not smoking. Put in the endives in a single layer. This is most efficiently done with the tips pointing toward the center. A few can go in the middle. Turn each endive over with tongs every 5 to 10 minutes so that they brown on all sides. It will take a good 30 minutes.

Pour the chicken stock over the endives. Cover the pan and turn the heat to low. Cook for about 1 hour or until a knife slips easily into the heavy end of an endive. They will not be mushy. Stir in salt and pepper to taste and serve.

SERVES 6 OR 7

CORN RELISH

I once gave the name "Corn of Plenty" to an article I wrote about corn because it provides us plentifully with animal feed, oil, dry ground grains for grits, masa, and polenta, and even fuel. In the summer it is in its full glory as a fresh vegetable. You can see the tassels turning russet and brown, letting you know the corn is ripe.

Sadly, it does not keep its natural sweetness for long when harvested. The sugar turns to starch. There are the supersweet corns, but I loathe them. They don't taste juicy and fresh. Unlike good standard corn, they are cloying and weary.

I eat as many quickly microwaved, steamed, boiled, baked, and grilled ears as even greed permits. They cook brilliantly in their husks when microwaved, baked—as in a clambake—or grilled. The husks preserve the moisture and add a fresh green flavor.

The kernels can be cut from the husks and added, raw or cooked, to salads and soups or combined with young lima beans to make succotash. The shucked ears can be cut across into 1-inch wedges to add to Central and South American soups and stews. Each row of kernels can be sliced lengthwise and then have the pulp scraped out with the back of a knife to make creamy soups and chowders.

After my appetite is satiated, it is time to think of the meals ahead. One of my favorite ways of keeping corn is in relish. The relish can be frozen or canned for the future.

3 cups golden corn kernels (from about 6 ears)

3 cups green cabbage in ½-inch squares (from about 1 small head)

1 cup finely chopped onion (from about 1 onion)

1 cup red bell pepper in ¼-inch squares (from about 2 large peppers)

1 cup green bell pepper in ¼-inch squares (from about 2 large peppers)

2 tablespoons prepared American brown mustard

3¾ cups white vinegar

2¼ cups sugar

3 tablespoons dry mustard

3 tablespoons kosher salt

2 heaping teaspoons hot red pepper flakes

1 tablespoon peeled and finely chopped ginger (about 6 quarter-sized pieces)

4 garlic cloves, smashed, peeled, and finely chopped

2 tablespoons arrowroot

Place all the ingredients, except ½ cup of the vinegar and the arrowroot, in a saucepan. Heat until the mixture just comes to a full simmer. Blend the arrowroot and reserved vinegar together and stir into the mixture. Remove from the heat, cool, and refrigerate for at least 24 hours for flavor to develop. Eat, can, or freeze in 1 pint amounts.

MAKES A GENEROUS 2 QUARTS

SAUTÉED CHARD

This is a simple way of preparing chard of any color. It can be multiplied as often as wanted and frozen in ½-cup amounts to use as a vegetable or in a soup.

1 tablespoon olive oil

1½ pounds chard with stems if tender or 1½ pounds leaves only, cut across into thin strips

Warm the oil in a large saucepan over medium heat. Gradually add the chard. After all the strips are in, cook for 10 minutes.

MAKES 1½ CUPS

VARIATION

Chard with Mashed Potatoes

Consider adding the chard to mashed potatoes—½ cup cooked chard to 4 cups mashed potatoes.

VAGUELY ASIAN EASY EGGPLANT

This is a gentle dish that went well with pork chops one evening. It is not so exotic that I didn't have the Sautéed Zucchini with Dill (page 154) on the same plate. In fact, a green of some kind is a good idea as the eggplant, although delicious, is drab to look at. I suppose that some chopped cilantro on top would not be amiss.

It may seem odd that I use a saucepan rather than a frying or sauté pan for this, but the eggplant shrinks so much that it is liable to burn in a pan of larger diameter.

¼ cup plus 1 teaspoon toasted sesame oil

1 large eggplant (about 1 pound), sliced in half lengthwise, then into 1-inch strips lengthwise and across into 1½-inch lengths

2 tablespoons gluten-free soy sauce

2 tablespoons mirin

1 tablespoon rice wine vinegar

Heat the oil in a 4-quart saucepan until shimmering but not smoking. Cook the eggplant, turning it with tongs from top to bottom. Do not stir or you will have mush. Allow it to color slightly. Add the soy, mirin, and vinegar and mix from time to time until the eggplant is tender.

SERVES 4 TO 6

RUBY CHARD STEMS AND ANCHOVY SAUTÉ

Ruby chard has green leaves but red stems and ribs. Its flavor is beetlike. Sautéeing the stems of ruby chard in an anchovy and garlic paste makes for a Mediterranean dish that is sweetened just a bit by raisins.

1 pound ruby chard stems (leaves reserved for another use), trimmed and cut across into ¾-inch pieces (about 4 cups)

¼ cup raisins

2 cloves garlic, smashed and peeled

1 teaspoon kosher salt

One 2-ounce can oil-packed flat anchovy fillets, rinsed

1 tablespoon fennel seeds

1 teaspoon olive oil

1 cup pulp from a large peeled tomato, seeded and chopped, or canned whole tomatoes, drained, squeezed, and roughly chopped

Freshly ground black pepper

Bring 10 cups water to a boil. Add the chard stems. Cover and cook over high heat until the water returns to a boil. Uncover and cook for 10 to 12 minutes. Strain in a colander, reserving ½ cup of liquid. Run the stems under cold water to refresh. Leave in the colander to drain for 10 to 15 minutes. May be prepared 3 to 4 hours ahead up to this point.

Soak the raisins in the reserved ½ cup liquid for 15 minutes.

In a mortar, crush the garlic with the kosher salt to make a paste. Add the anchovies and fennel seeds. Crush until fairly smooth. Place the raisins with the liquid in a microwave oven and cook for 1 minute or simmer on top of the stove until softened. Drain the raisins.

In a medium saucepan, combine the olive oil with the blanched stems, garlic-anchovy paste, raisins, tomato pulp, and pepper to taste. Cook over low heat, stirring, until warmed through.

SERVES 4 TO 6

GRILLED MUSHROOMS

I often make these to accompany the Grilled Flank Steak (page 106).

> About ½ cup olive oil for every pound of mushrooms
>
> Kosher salt
>
> Freshly ground black pepper
>
> Portobello mushrooms, stemmed and wiped clean of dirt with a damp paper towel

Preheat a grill until quite hot. Combine the oil in a bowl with salt and pepper to taste. Turn the mushrooms in the oil until well coated. Place around the edges of the grill, top side down. Longer-cooking vegetables, meat, or fish can be cooked over the central, hottest part of the grill.

The length of time needed to cook the mushrooms will depend on the heat of the fire and the size of the mushrooms. When the mushrooms are about half cooked, brush the underside with oil and turn over. Brush any remaining oil over the skins as required and continue grilling until cooked through. Remove from the grill and season with salt and pepper to taste.

SERVES 5 OR 6

LARGE LIMA BEANS SIMMERED WITH ONION AND GARLIC

Good with a salad of any sort or as a side to roasted or grilled meats.

> 2 cups dried large lima beans
>
> ¼ pound white onion, cut into chunks (about 1 cup)
>
> 2 large cloves garlic, smashed and peeled
>
> 2 tablespoons olive oil
>
> 4 cups vegetable broth (homemade, page 206, or good commercial stock)
>
> Large pinch dried sage leaves, crumbled
>
> ½ teaspoon dried thyme
>
> 2 teaspoons kosher salt
>
> Freshly ground black pepper

Soak the beans in plenty of skin-temperature water overnight.

Chop the onion and garlic in a food processor until the onion is very finely chopped. Heat the olive oil in a medium skillet. Add the onion mixture and cook until the onion is translucent, about 4 minutes.

Scrape the onion mixture into a slow cooker. Drain the beans and add to the slow cooker. Add the stock and enough water to cover the beans by an inch (about 2 cups). Stir in the sage and thyme.

Cook on low heat for 8 hours, until the beans are tender and the liquid just covers them. If there is too much liquid, transfer the beans to a serving bowl. Tilt the slow cooker and ladle the liquid into a saucepan. Bring to a boil and cook until there is just enough liquid to cover the beans.

Stir in salt and pepper to taste, and serve.

MAKES 4 TO 5 CUPS

KWIK KALE

I tend to do things the way I have always done them; but looking at the mountain of kale in my kitchen, I thought there had to be a better way than removing the stems and cutting them across in thinnish strips, to sauté, steam, and purée if desired. This recipe is my quick and easy solution. A little salt turns it into a good vegetable.

> 3 to 4 large bunches kale, stemmed and coarsely chopped
> 2 tablespoons olive oil
> Kosher salt

Working in batches, put the kale leaves in a food processor and process until they are very finely chopped. There should be about 4½ cups. Place the kale and olive oil in a large saucepan and cook for 45 minutes over medium heat. Season with salt to taste.

MAKES 3 CUPS

VARIATION

Kwik Kale Soup
Two cups cooked Kwik Kale plus 2½ cups stock makes this a good soup. If not thick enough, stir in 2½ teaspoons arrowroot or potato starch that's been mixed with 1½ tablespoons cold water to make a slurry.

SERVES 4 TO 6

SWEET AND SOUR LENTILS

Many green vegetables—beans, chopped spinach, Brussels sprouts, and the tops of broccoli—profit from being mixed with some white vinegar and brown sugar, in equal proportions. Slivered almonds on top of the dishes add élan.

This sweet and sour dish, which is made with lentils, takes a little longer to prepare but is worth the trouble because no one leaving your house is going to meet it the next day at someone else's.

> 1½ cups dried brown lentils
> 1 medium onion, cut into ¼-inch dice
> 4 cups Extra-Rich Chicken Stock (page 204)
> 2 tablespoons chicken fat or olive oil
> ½ teaspoon kosher salt
> ¼ teaspoon coarsely ground black pepper
> Juice of 1 lemon
> 2 tablespoons sugar
> Paprika

Boil the lentils and onion in the stock for 45 minutes, until tender. Drain the liquid into another pot. Put the fat in a casserole over medium heat, and add the salt, pepper, lemon juice, and sugar. Cook for 1 minute, then add ½ cup of the reserved stock. Can be made in advance to this point.

Heat the oven to 350°F.

Add the lentils to the casserole. Put in the oven and bake for 15 minutes (20 minutes if made in advance). Sprinkle with paprika and serve. This dish can be made in advance, except for the baking, and then heated in the oven for 20 minutes.

MAKES 4 CUPS

RED CABBAGE, ITALIAN VARIATION

This is a typically sweet and sour dish that I usually think of as German or Russian. I was making it to go with roast duck (see page 98). Gazing around the kitchen while thinly slicing the cabbage I sighted a bottle of balsamic vinegar. I had an "aha" moment. Why not use it as both the sweet and the sour? It worked perfectly and required no added sugar. I substituted anise seeds for the usual caraway and found it an improvement.

> ¼ cup olive oil
>
> 2 red onions (about 1 pound), thinly sliced (about 3 cups)
>
> Large head red cabbage, halved through the stem end, cored, and thinly sliced across (15 to 16 cups)
>
> ⅓ cup balsamic vinegar
>
> 2 tablespoons anise seeds
>
> Kosher salt (optional)

Heat the oil in a heavy pot large enough to hold all the ingredients (10 to 11 inches across). Add the onions and cook over medium heat, stirring, for about 5 minutes. Add the cabbage and cook for 20 minutes more, stirring from top to bottom. Add the vinegar and cook for 20 minutes. Stir in the anise seeds and cook for 10 minutes. Taste and add salt if desired.

MAKES 9 TO 10 CUPS

RUTABAGA TAMED

I have never liked rutabaga. Recently, however, a blog friend pointed out that it was a great favorite in German-speaking countries. I determined to try again. I tried to order small ones; instead, I received two that weighed 3 pounds each. To peel them, I had to take a heavy knife, push it into the stem ends, and cut across by picking up the knife and joined vegetable together and smacking them hard onto the butcher block. That got rid of all four ends.

Then I took a sharp new vegetable peeler and peeled. I repeated the smashing technique to cut each one into quarters. At that point it was easy to cut them across into ¼-inch slices. There were 16 cups that I put into a very large pot and covered with water and a lid. After bringing the rutabaga to a boil, I cooked it for 20 minutes, until I could slip in a knife. I tasted it and still didn't like it. Then the fun began. It became delicious.

> 16 cups sliced rutabaga, prepared and cooked as described above
>
> ½ cup olive oil, or more as needed
>
> 1 cup coarsely chopped soft tips of a very large bunch dill
>
> 2 tablespoons kosher salt

Drain the rutabaga and purée through the fine disc of a food mill. Combine well with the oil, dill, and salt. If it seems dry, add more olive oil to taste. Stirring well, heat for 20 minutes when ready to serve.

MAKES 8 CUPS; SERVES 12

VARIATION

Tamed Rutabaga Soup

Reserve the broth as you drain the rutabaga. After thinning to the desired consistency with more broth, this dish is an excellent soup, serving 15 people.

DEEP-ROASTED FALL VEGETABLES

These are not al dente crisp vegetables. These are browned, intensely flavored, and fully cooked until soft.

> 3 tablespoons olive oil or safflower oil
>
> 1 pound small white onions (about 1¼ inches in diameter), peeled
>
> ½ pound small to medium carrots, peeled and cut across into 1-inch slices—larger carrots should be halved lengthwise (about 1 cup)
>
> 1 bunch broccoli, cut into small florets (about 4 cups)
>
> 1 pound yellow summer squash—not zucchini—quartered lengthwise and cut into 1-inch pieces (about 4 cups)
>
> 2 tablespoons chopped fresh marjoram leaves (optional)
>
> Kosher salt
>
> Freshly ground black pepper

Heat the oven to 500°F with a rack at the lowest level.

Put the oil into a 14-×-18-×-2-inch or slightly smaller roasting pan. Swirl the oil so it coats the bottom of the pan. Put in the onions and shake so that they are coated. Roast for 10 minutes. Shake to turn over. Move the onions to the center of the pan and surround with the remaining vegetables. Roast for 15 minutes. Turn over. Roast for 15 minutes longer. If using marjoram, add it 3 minutes before the end of the roasting time.

Season with salt and pepper to taste and serve hot. If serving tepid or cool, add a little more olive oil and a little balsamic vinegar.

MAKES 4 CUPS

TURNIP ROAST

Heat the oven to 500°F with the rack in the center. Use 1 medium to large turnip per person. Peel and cut each into 6 wedges. Rub on all sides with safflower oil—about 2 teaspoons for each turnip. Roast for about 30 minutes, shaking twice to turn the wedges. They will be lightly, spottily browned. Serve immediately.

WONDERFUL TURNIP MASH

I never used to be a lover of turnips, but since I discovered mashing them on their own—not with potatoes—I have been converted. I prefer the white kind, the best being Gilfeather. Gilfeather is a farm up near me in Vermont, and these turnips are milder in taste and less fibrous than most. If you can, try to get seed and grow them. They like the cold; I pull them in late fall. Like winter squash, they will keep for a long time, or they can be made as in this recipe and frozen; they will take less room. Gilfeathers can get huge—1½ to 2 pounds. Mashed, they don't serve that many.

> 1½ pounds white turnips, peeled and cut into 1-inch cubes (see Note)
>
> 1 tablespoon olive oil
>
> 1 teaspoon kosher salt

Put 4 cups cold water in the bottom of a steamer. Lay the turnip cubes in the steamer basket and cover. Bring the water to a boil and cook for 20 minutes. Put through the medium disc of a food mill. There will be about 2 cups. Reheat when ready to eat; stir in the olive oil and salt.

SERVES 4

NOTE

It may be necessary to make a cut in the peeled turnip and—with the knife in the cut—slam the turnip and knife onto a cutting board.

SWEETLY TASTY TURNIPS

Turnips can vary. This is a somewhat unusual recipe for the ordinary white and purple turnips. I developed it for a friend who is a vegan. It is a real sign of friendship to create meals for vegans. Turnips can be rather acrid, but not in this preparation. It is a good addition to a vegan assortment or as a side dish for fish or smoked meat. The recipe can be doubled.

> 1 pound turnips, peeled, cut into quarters, and thinly sliced
>
> ½ cup mirin
>
> ¼ cup rice wine vinegar
>
> 2 tablespoons toasted sesame oil
>
> Kosher salt
>
> Freshly ground black pepper

Combine the turnips, mirin, vinegar, and sesame oil in a medium saucepan. Bring to a boil and cover. Reduce the heat and simmer for about 40 minutes or until the turnips are cooked but not mushy. Season with salt and pepper to taste. The turnips may not need additional salt and pepper. Serve drained, using the cooking liquid to cook other mild vegetables or fish or white meat of chicken.

SERVES 4

VARIATION

Sort-of Caesar Dressing

The leftover liquid also makes an excellent salad dressing, mixed two parts to one with mayonnaise. I used about ½ cup liquid and cut 3 hard-boiled eggs into the mixture. It doesn't make up for missing out on Caesar salad, but it is a substantial and satisfying dressing.

ACORN SQUASH PURÉE

Good, simple, and colorful with any roast.

> 1 acorn squash (about 2 pounds), cut in half through the stem and seeded
>
> ⅓ cup coconut milk
>
> Pinch cayenne pepper
>
> Kosher salt

Place the squash halves, cut side up, on a large platter. Cover tightly with plastic wrap and microwave on high for 10 minutes. Pierce the plastic with the tip of a sharp knife to release steam. Scoop the flesh out of the halves and place in a food processor with the coconut milk. Purée until the mixture is completely smooth, 3 to 4 minutes. Season with the cayenne and salt to taste.

MAKES 2½ CUPS

MEAL BUILDERS

We Intolerants can eat this group of starch recipes with impunity. I think they are terrific and I hope they encourage invention and the use of some unfamiliar foods.

GARLIC MASHED POTATOES

I have always loved mashed potatoes. As a child, I would make a hollow in my mound of potatoes and fill it with gravy. I thought that pleasure was over forever. Well, I have come up with a version of mashed potatoes without butter or cream. I didn't believe they could be this good.

I have tried using various kinds of potatoes. The least good have been those I used to use—the Idahos, russets, and Maine or boiling potatoes. By far the best are potatoes without too much starch. The clue to trying them came from superstar chef Joël Robuchon. He was named "chef of the century" in 1990, has twenty-six Michelin stars (more than any other chef in the world), and makes the most fabulous mashed potatoes I've ever had. His are made with Rattes, a variety of waxy potato that originated in the north of France and is still popular with French chefs. I don't claim that these are the equal of Robuchon's; but they are very good and have the advantage that they can be reheated, unlike his, which are made at the last minute (if you are fortunate enough to dine at one of his restaurants and see the kitchen, be sure to look for the poor cook whose sole task is to make mashed potatoes all night long).

Don't make the garlic oil too far ahead or reduce the amount of garlic.

This recipe can easily be doubled, and the potatoes reheat fairly well (even days later), though they will not be as tasty as freshly made. The garlic flavor also gets stronger with time. SEE COLOR PLATE 16

12 cloves garlic, smashed, peeled, and cut into ⅛-inch slices

½ cup olive oil

2 pounds red or fingerling potatoes, peeled and cut into 1-inch chunks (about 4 cups)

Kosher salt

Place the garlic and oil in a small saucepan over very low heat.

In a medium saucepan, bring 2 quarts water to a boil. Add the potatoes and reduce the heat to simmer. Cook for 10 to 12 minutes or until the tip of a sharp knife easily pierces a potato. Drain. Place the potatoes back in the pot to dry out for 2 minutes.

Pass the potatoes through a food mill fitted with the fine disc into a large bowl. Strain the garlic oil into the potatoes. Mix with a whisk and season with salt to taste.

MAKES 1 SCANT QUART; SERVES 4 TO 6 AS A SIDE DISH

VARIATION

Olive Oil Mashed Potatoes

Omit the garlic.

SCALLION DUCK RICE

This is yet another reason to enjoy the stock that comes from roasting duck. It can, of course, be served with a grilled duck breast; but, oddly, it goes very well with a simple fish or chicken.

> 3 cups cooked black rice (see page 228)
>
> 1 cup duck stock, or more if needed (see page 98; use chicken stock if duck is unavailable)
>
> 1 bunch scallions (about 4 ounces), trimmed and cut across into ¼-inch slices (1½ cups)
>
> 2 teaspoons Lemon Zesty Spice Mix (page 202)
>
> Kosher salt
>
> Freshly ground black pepper

Place the cooked black rice with the duck stock in a medium saucepan over high heat. Bring to a boil, reduce the heat to simmer, and cook for 5 minutes. Add the scallions and spice mixture, turn the heat to medium, and stir well. If the rice appears dry, add more duck stock as needed. Season with salt and pepper to taste.

MAKES 1 SCANT QUART; SERVES 4

BUCKWHEAT WITH VEGETABLES

Poor buckwheat has gotten a bad reputation due to the "wheat" in its name. In fact it is not a wheat at all, but rather a nutty-tasting grain known to Jews as "kasha." It is a wonderful accompaniment with almost all full-tasting meats, from beef and pork to quail, venison, and squab.

> 2 cups chicken stock (any of the homemade stocks, pages 203–4, or sterile-pack)
>
> 1 bay leaf
>
> 1 cup buckwheat (kasha)
>
> 1 tablespoon safflower oil
>
> 1 small onion, minced (about ½ cup)
>
> 4 large mushrooms, trimmed and cut into ⅛-inch dice (about 1 cup)
>
> 2 large stalks celery, peeled and cut into ⅛-inch dice (about ½ cup)
>
> Kosher salt
>
> Freshly ground black pepper

Put the chicken stock and bay leaf in a 3-quart stockpot and bring to a boil. Add the buckwheat, reduce the heat to simmer, cover, and cook for 8 minutes.

Heat the oil in an 8-inch sauté pan over medium-low heat. Sauté the onion until soft, 2 to 3 minutes. Add the mushrooms and celery and continue cooking for 3 minutes. When the buckwheat is fully cooked, stir in the vegetables. Season with salt and pepper to taste.

MAKES 3⅓ CUPS; SERVES 6

CHESTNUT AND WALNUT DRESSING

This is a dressing, not a stuffing, as it doesn't go inside the bird. It is delicious and is a justification for the idea of progress in food—even packaged food. It is now possible to buy jars of peeled, roasted chestnuts, unsweetened. Chestnuts have long been an ingredient in stuffing for fowl, but here they are the main component. Turkey stock will give a sense of a stuffing, if available. Chicken stock can also be used, and if water replaces stock, it is a perfect dish for vegetarians or vegans at the feast.

This recipe can be doubled using an ordinary food processor. The only fiddly parts are chopping the leaves and dicing the peeled celery. Add salt carefully. Celery is really very salty.

1 pound celery stalks

1 large bunch parsley, stemmed

One 15-ounce jar peeled, roasted chestnuts, more or less

¼ cup chestnut flour

¾ cup turkey stock, chicken stock (any of the homemade stocks, pages 203–4, or sterile-pack), water, or apple juice

Kosher salt

Freshly ground black pepper

½ cup walnut pieces

Peel the celery stalks and reserve the leaves. Cut the stalks into ¼-inch dice and set aside. Coarsely chop the parsley and celery leaves; lightly packed, there should be about ½ cup.

Pulse the chestnuts in a food processor until coarsely chopped. From time to time, scrape down the sides of the bowl with a spatula. In a very small saucepan, whisk together the chestnut flour and stock until there are no lumps. Cook over very low heat, whisking until slightly thickened. Scrape into the chestnuts. Add the chopped leaves and diced celery. Process just until mixed. Taste for salt and pepper. Add the walnut pieces and process just until mixed.

The dressing can be made ahead and reheated on top of the stove, in a microwave, or in a regular oven, wherever space can be found. It doesn't need cooking, just heating, and I think it actually improves with a day or two of aging.

MAKES 3 CUPS

QUINOA

This good-to-eat seed (grain) that I often serve as a side dish, or as a replacement for rice when I want a risotto but am short on time, is a nutritional wonder.

To cook quinoa, use twice as much liquid as quinoa by volume (2 cups water to 1 cup quinoa, for example). I usually add a little olive oil to the water. It can also be seasoned when cooked.

Bring the liquid to a boil. Add the quinoa. Stir and reduce the heat so that the quinoa bubbles. It will take from 15 to 20 minutes to cook, depending on the heat.

Recipes like Ultimate Quinoa for Fish and Chicken (opposite) use more liquid, which is not a mistake. The added ingredients require it.

QUINOA WITH CELERY AND MUSHROOMS

I can just hear someone shouting "Oh, no, not quinoa again," but this is really good. I made it for friends who cannot eat onions or garlic. Looking around for a solution, I found that the freezer had two plastic containers of *Boletus* mushrooms that I had picked, cooked, and frozen in the summer. If—as is probable—fresh *Boletus* are not available, use another good mushroom. Even if you don't forage as I do, you will find an expanding selection of flavorful mushrooms in shops—labeled "wild" only to differentiate them from regular mushrooms. Prepare as on pages 208–9. They need not be frozen. In fact, they will need to be defrosted if frozen.

Don't worry if this makes more than you need. My friends took home the remains, and so will yours. SEE COLOR PLATE 8

> 3 cups chicken stock (**any of the homemade stocks, pages 203–4, or sterile-pack**)
>
> 1½ cups quinoa
>
> 3 medium stalks celery, peeled and cut into ¼-inch dice (about 1 cup), leaves reserved
>
> 1 cup wild mushrooms, cut into pieces and cooked (see pages 208–9)
>
> ½ cup lightly packed celery leaves, finely chopped
>
> Kosher salt
>
> Freshly ground black pepper

In a medium saucepan, bring the stock to a boil over high heat. Add the quinoa and diced celery, return to a boil, reduce the heat to simmer, cover, and cook for 12 to 14 minutes. Stir in the mushrooms, cook for 1 to 2 minutes, and stir in the celery leaves. Season with salt and pepper to taste.

MAKES ABOUT 7 CUPS

ULTIMATE QUINOA FOR FISH AND CHICKEN

As good as quinoa is as a healthful nutty grain on its own, there are times when a little gussying up is a welcome idea, especially with milder-tasting main courses such as fish and chicken. A liberal dose of vegetables, a change in liquid, and some herbs do the trick. Choose your stock or stock mixture according to what the quinoa is being served with. I used half fish and half chicken to go with black bass, a mild-tasting fish. Each fish served two. There was some leftover quinoa, which in my continuous kitchen mode is very nice the next day for lunch or as a starter.

> 1½ cups Fish Stock (page 205)
>
> 1½ cups chicken stock (any of the homemade stocks, pages 203–4, or sterile-pack)
>
> 2 teaspoons kosher salt
>
> 1½ cups quinoa
>
> 6 ounces red onion, cut into ¼-inch cubes (about ¾ cup)
>
> 6 ounces mild white onion, cut into ¼-inch cubes (about ¾ cup)
>
> 2 medium cucumbers, peeled, seeded, and cut into ¼-inch cubes (about ¾ cup)
>
> ¾ cup finely chopped dill, or ¾ cup lovage or flat-leaf parsley thinly sliced across
>
> 2 tablespoons fresh lemon juice
>
> Kosher salt
>
> Freshly ground black pepper
>
> Olive oil (optional)

Bring the stocks to a boil. Stir in the salt and quinoa. Reduce the heat to a low boil. Cook for 10 minutes. Add the onions and cook for 5 minutes. If need be, add water. Add the cucumbers, dill, and lemon juice. Season with salt and pepper to taste. Serve hot or warm or at room temperature in the latter case, toss with olive oil to taste.

SERVES 6 TO 8

TEFF

Teff will probably have to be ordered online, but it's worth it. This flour cooks quickly and makes an all-purpose side dish that takes well to one's favorite seasonings. Think of it as a rapid polenta.

BASIC TEFF

This side dish uses the tiny teff grains ground into a flour (for more information, see page 232). It is increasingly available in stores. The flavor will be slightly nutty—not strange.

> ½ cup teff flour
>
> Kosher salt

Bring 1½ cups water to a boil in a small saucepan. Whisk the teff flour into ½ cup cold water, then whisk the mixture into the boiling water until well combined. Reduce the heat to simmer and cook for 3 to 4 minutes, stirring occasionally. Season with salt to taste.

MAKES 2 CUPS

TEFF TO YOUR TASTE

Teff can be made into an alternative to mashed potatoes or polenta that's a pleasing nut brown. Cook carefully to avoid lumps.

One intelligent friend said this would make a good breakfast. I don't eat much in the morning, but leftovers would be a good start to the day. Try slicing a banana on top.

    Kosher salt
    2 tablespoons safflower oil
    2½ tablespoons ground cumin
    1½ cups teff flour
    One 14-ounce can coconut milk
    Freshly ground black pepper

Combine 4 cups water, 2 tablespoons kosher salt, the safflower oil, and the cumin. Bring to a simmer. Beating with a whisk, pour in the teff flour. Beating constantly, bring to a low boil. Add the coconut milk. When thickened, remove from the heat and continue to beat until smooth. If there are lumps, purée in a food processor. Taste for salt and pepper. Reheat carefully.

MAKES 5½ CUPS, PLENTY FOR 6

POLENTA

There are many variations of the preparation of corn; some of them are on pages 220–21. Polenta with Oregano and Olive Oil is a special favorite.

SOFT POLENTA

For corn and polenta basics, see pages 219–21. We gave the Italians corn, and they returned the favor, with polenta. It replaced the millet that the Roman army had used. Soft, it is an ideal side dish or base for stews.

    ¾ cup yellow or white cornmeal
    2 teaspoons kosher salt
    3 tablespoons olive oil
    ⅛ teaspoon freshly ground pepper

Combine 4 cups water with the cornmeal and salt in a 2-quart soufflé dish. Cook, uncovered, in a microwave oven on high for 6 minutes. Stir well, cover loosely with paper toweling, and cook for 6 minutes more.

Remove from the oven. Uncover and stir in the olive oil and pepper. Let stand for 3 minutes. Serve hot.

MAKES 5½ CUPS; SERVES 8 AS A SIDE DISH

VARIATIONS

Soft Polenta for One or Two
Quarter all the ingredients (use 3 tablespoons cornmeal). Proceed as directed, cooking in a soup bowl for 1 minute and 30 seconds, uncovered, and then for another 1 minute and 30 seconds, covered.

Soft Polenta for Three or Four
Combine 2½ cups water, ½ cup cornmeal, and 1 teaspoon salt in an 8-cup glass measure. Cook as directed for 5 minutes. Stir and continue to cook for 5 minutes longer. Finish as directed, stirring in 2 tablespoons olive oil and a pinch of pepper.

POLENTA WITH OREGANO AND OLIVE OIL

Polenta is the name Italy gave cornmeal when the country adopted it. The polenta can be firm (recipe follows) or creamy, as here, where it makes a wonderful accompaniment to almost anything—even stews that are a little thin like one I made by poaching chicken thighs with cut-up chanterelles. No recipe for that because I am afraid to tell anyone how to forage. But if you can get store-bought chanterelles, three skinned thighs will take a cup of cut-up mushrooms and enough chicken broth to cover. I find myself eating the polenta on its own—even cool.

> 5½ cups Soft Polenta (preceding recipe)
> 1 bunch oregano, stemmed and roughly chopped (2 tablespoons packed)
> ¼ cup olive oil
> ⅛ teaspoon freshly ground black pepper
> Kosher salt

Mix all the ingredients except the salt together. Season with salt to taste. The polenta can be refrigerated and then reheats well over low heat with stirring.

MAKES 5½ CUPS

FIRM POLENTA

Firm polenta is usually made, allowed to cool, and then cut into pieces for sautéing or grilling.

> 1¼ cups yellow or white cornmeal
> 2 teaspoons kosher salt
> ¼ cup olive oil
> ⅛ teaspoon freshly ground pepper

Combine 4 cups water with the cornmeal and salt in a 2-quart soufflé dish. Cook, uncovered, in a microwave on high for 11 minutes, stirring once.

Remove from the oven, stir in 3 tablespoons of the oil, and add the pepper. Let stand for 3 minutes.

Lightly grease a 7-x-4-x-2-inch loaf pan with half the remaining tablespoon of olive oil. Pour the polenta into the pan and brush lightly with the last of the oil. Let stand until cool.

Cover and refrigerate until chilled. To serve, slice the polenta about ½ inch thick and fry or grill.

SERVES 8 AS PART OF A FIRST COURSE OR AS A SIDE DISH

DESSERTS

I have never been a big eater of desserts. My husband and many of my friends like to end a meal with something sweet. In reality, I think some of them—like many small children—consider the rest of the meal a foreword to the dessert.

This is not a baking book. There are a few baking recipes here; but I do think that I have created enough delicious and special recipes that the more conventional cakes and tarts will not be missed.

There are "ice creams" and sorbets at the end of the chapter.

Do take a look at the sauces on pages 198–99 and the superior waffle on page 16 as well.

LIGHTEST MERINGUES

I love meringues, and as they have no gluten or lactose they are a perfect snack for me. I don't like them gooey or overly sweet and am uninterested in the fancy colored ones that have recently cropped up in the fancy pastry shops and French restaurants. I hope you will find these, which I developed recently, as addictive as I do. These are the meringues that I use lightly crushed to coat chunks of ripe but firm banana as a seduction.

4 egg whites, at room temperature
¼ cup sugar

Preheat the oven to 150°F with two racks inside. Cover each of two cookie sheets with a layer of parchment paper. Have ready a pastry bag with a ½-inch-diameter nozzle and set aside.

Place the egg whites in an electric mixer with a stainless-steel bowl and start to beat them slowly. Beat until frothy. Pour in the sugar and continue to beat. Increase the speed to the fullest. Beat until the egg whites are very stiff—when they hold stiff peaks.

Now move quickly or the mixture will not stay ideally firm: Spoon the stiff egg whites into the pastry bag. Squeeze out 2-inch-long strips of meringue onto the baking sheets so that they do not touch. Place both baking sheets in the oven and cook for 1½ hours.

Turn off the oven and leave the meringues undisturbed for about another hour. They should be crisp and dry without being colored. Remove the baking sheets from the oven and slide the meringues, still on their paper, onto a flat surface. Allow the meringues to cool to room temperature. Slide a metal spatula or thin ham slicer under the meringues to remove them from the paper.

Eat or store the meringues in an airtight box.

MAKES ABOUT 54 MERINGUES

MOCHA MERINGUES

These can be enjoyed alone or made into a layered dessert using the Chocolate Marsala Pudding (page 178) in between the meringue layers. The meringue can also be made into a savory snack; see Spicy Kisses (page 29).

4 egg whites, at room temperature
⅓ cup sugar
1 teaspoon instant espresso powder
1 teaspoon unsweetened cocoa powder

Preheat the oven to 250°F with one rack at the top and another in the middle. Cover each of two 12-×-15-inch cookie sheets with a layer of parchment paper. Have ready a pastry bag with a ½-inch-diameter nozzle and set aside.

Place the egg whites in an electric mixer and start to beat slowly. Beat until frothy. Slowly add the sugar. Increase the speed to the fullest. Beat until the egg whites are very stiff—when they hold stiff peaks. Fold in the espresso and cocoa powder.

Now move quickly or the mixture will not stay ideally firm: Spoon the stiff egg whites into the pastry bag. Either form as and cook as in the preceding recipe or use as a layer in a dacquoise.

Turn off the oven and leave the meringues undisturbed for 1½ hours. They should be crisp and dry. Remove the baking sheets from the oven and slide the meringues, still on their paper, onto a flat surface. Slide a metal spatula or thin ham slicer under the meringues to remove them from the paper. Eat or store the meringues in an airtight box.

MAKES ABOUT 54 MERINGUES

AMARETTI WOLSELEY

Many times in my career I have asked chefs for recipes— mostly without results. However, when good friends took me to lunch at the Wolseley restaurant on Piccadilly in London, I asked the pastry chef, Regis Negrier, for his recipe for amaretti. Much to my pleased surprise, the recipe arrived a week or so later by e-mail.

I felt like an idiot for not having thought of making amaretti for this book; but the chagrin was worth it. These are not your usual crisp, dry Italian kind but a truly luscious invention by a German chef, much more like macaroons. I had to modify the recipe slightly since his used prepared marzipan paste. Both it and the American almond paste available in tubes cannot be used due to the presence of wheat. I think that this variation is just about as good as the original.

1¾ cups slivered blanched almonds

3 tablespoons light corn syrup

¾ cup confectioners' sugar

1 egg white, at room temperature

1 tablespoon dried figs in ⅛-inch dice (1 to 2 whole figs)

1 tablespoon dried apricots in ⅛-inch dice (2 to 3 whole apricots)

1 tablespoon dried cranberries in ⅛-inch dice

Put the almonds, corn syrup, ¼ cup plus 1 tablespoon of the confectioners' sugar, and the egg white in a food processor and process for 3 to 4 minutes, until well combined or the mixture looks like fine wet sand. Using a spatula, scrape the contents into a bowl and add the dried fruit. Mix well. Divide the mixture into 12 pieces and roll each piece into a ball using the palms of your hands. Roll the balls around in the remaining confectioners' sugar until fully coated, then place them on a nonstick baking sheet.

Let the amaretti dry for at least an hour. Heat the oven to 400°F with a rack in the top third. Bake the amaretti for 10 minutes or until golden brown. Remove from the oven and allow to cool.

MAKES 12 AMARETTI

ORANGE-POACHED FIGS

The purple, brown, or black fresh figs you find in America are actually the same variety but in different states of ripeness. Despite their unromantic name—Brown Turkeys—these figs are the most like the Mediterranean variety and are particularly good with rich meats and in desserts with creamy sauces. At their ripest in the fall—in the black stage—they tend to be fragile but richer in flavor. Use them in sauces or with ham. The purple or brown figs hold their shape better, so they are best for salads or eating out of hand.

These figs would welcome the Zabaglione (page 199).

12 medium or 16 small fresh black figs (¾ pound), stemmed

¼ cup sugar

⅛ teaspoon freshly ground black pepper

One 2-inch piece vanilla bean, split lengthwise

⅜ cup fresh orange juice

3 tablespoons fresh lemon juice

2 tablespoons Marsala (optional)

Place the figs upright in a saucepan just large enough to hold them comfortably in one layer. Sprinkle with the sugar and pepper. Add the vanilla bean and the juices over the figs.

Cover the pan and slowly bring to a boil over medium heat. Lower the temperature and simmer very gently for 10 to 15 minutes for medium figs, 5 to 10 minutes for small, or until cooked through but not falling apart. Add the Marsala, if desired, and stir. Serve warm.

SERVES 4

RHUBARB MISTAKE

Oddly, some of my favorite recipe ideas have come from mistakes. Of course, some mistakes have just yielded inedible messes. Over one weekend I got lucky. There was a flourish of rhubarb in the garden as part of the jungle that all the rain had produced. I sawed off—a bread knife works well—a few handfuls of stalks, discarding the poisonous leaves. I washed them, cut out the nasty bits, and trimmed off the root ends. I cut the stalks into ½-inch lengths and put them in a pot with sugar, mixed them up, and set them to cook. In the meantime I went back to the computer and forgot my rhubarb.

By the time I remembered, the mess was medium brown, and I had to poke and scrape to get the caramelized bits off the bottom and out of the corners. I was about to discard it when I stuck a finger in and took a small taste. To my shock and delight it was delicious. Consequently I have made it into a recipe. It's worth trying. Stir and be a little more careful than I was. (If you have trouble cleaning the pot, try scouring it with coarse salt.) It makes a great dessert with a splash of coconut milk.

½ pound rhubarb, trimmed, peeled, and cut into 1-inch lengths (about 4 cups)

¾ cup sugar

Put the rhubarb and sugar into a 6-inch stainless-steel saucepan. Stir thoroughly. Set over medium heat for 5 minutes or until all the sugar is dissolved. If you are nervous about it scorching, add ½ cup water. Stir and cook at a slow boil for about 45 minutes, stirring from time to time. If there is a lot of water—there should be some juice—boil to dry slightly. That's it.

MAKES 1½ CUPS; SERVES 6

COCONUT CUSTARD WITH AGAVE NECTAR

Thorny, horny cactus hardly leaps to mind as a food. We have come to think of its distilled juices, tequila (made from agave) and—even better—mezcal, as ingredients in cold, fruity, and delightful drinks, although very good aged mezcal (made from maguey cactus) is perhaps better drunk on its own like a good Scotch or brandy.

However, prepared prickly pear cactus (agave) pads readily available in cans have been one of the great benefits of the explosion of Mexican immigration to the United States. The pads are commonly served in salads (see page 67). They should be washed before use.

Agave nectar has been slower to make its way north of the border. It is a sweet syrup that can be used to replace sugar and honey.

Many health claims have been made for these cactus products, including their miraculous ability to cure a hangover.

This dessert is cool, white, and sweet—a make-ahead summertime pleasure. What is more, the contents can be kept on the shelf. The amaranth seeds are optional but attractive.

> 2 tablespoons plus 2 teaspoons powdered gelatin
>
> 2 cups coconut milk
>
> ½ teaspoon amaranth seeds (optional)
>
> 4 teaspoons agave nectar

Dissolve the gelatin in 1 cup of the coconut milk. Heat the mixture in a small saucepan until the gelatin is completely dissolved, less than a minute. Whisk the warm coconut milk into the remaining 1 cup coconut milk. Pour the mixture into a 7- or 8-inch square baking pan.

Refrigerate until firm to the touch, about 2 hours.

Place a 10-inch skillet over high heat. Allow the pan to get hot (a hand held over the pan should feel the heat) and scatter the amaranth evenly over the pan. The grains should start popping almost immediately and will increase in size and turn bright white. Set the popped amaranth aside.

Cut the coconut custard into cubes, and divide them evenly among four small bowls. Drizzle 1 teaspoon agave nectar and scatter some popped amaranth over each portion.

SERVES 4

CHOCOLATE MARSALA PUDDING

This satisfying pudding owes its silky smooth texture to the same principles as classic mayonnaise. The chocolate and Marsala add a deep, rich flavor that's not too sweet. I use half a recipe as filling between discs of Mocha Meringues (page 174). Using a chocolate with a higher cacao content will result in a more bitter pudding.

> 1½ cups safflower oil
>
> 2¼ ounces shaved (grated) 70% dark (not milk) chocolate
>
> ⅓ cup sugar
>
> 3 egg yolks
>
> ¼ cup dry Marsala

Warm the oil in a 2-cup glass measure in the microwave for 30 seconds. Dissolve the chocolate and sugar in the oil. Place the yolks in a food processor and mix until well blended. With the machine running, add the oil in a thin stream and process until thoroughly incorporated and the mixture is smooth. Add the Marsala and mix until just combined.

MAKES 2 GENEROUS CUPS

YUM YUM NUT SWEETS

I'm surprised and delighted by the number of sweets and desserts that I have been able to come up with sans flour and dairy. With this one I had help. Our good friend Dr. Nersessian—a very good cook—came up with the first version of this to give me a dessert without the bad things. I have fiddled with it a bit. It has been a great success with all who have tasted it. A chocolate version follows.

> ½ teaspoon safflower oil
>
> 1 cup whole roasted unsalted almonds
>
> 1 cup whole walnuts
>
> ⅓ cup sugar
>
> 2 egg whites

Preheat the oven to 300°F. Grease a 7- or 8-inch square baking pan with the oil. Set aside. Place the nuts in a food processor and chop until the mixture resembles coarse sand. Put the contents into a small mixing bowl. Stir in the sugar and egg whites. With a spatula, scrape the contents of the bowl into the oiled pan and press into an even layer. Bake for 1 hour for soft cookies or 1½ hours for crisp cookies. Remove from the oven. Allow to cool. Cut into 1¾- or 2-inch squares.

MAKES 16 SQUARES

VARIATION

Chocolate Yum Yums
Even though these are simply a chocolate version of the Yum Yums, everyone seems to think that they are brownies. Yum.

Melt 2½ ounces of 70% dark—not milk—chocolate in a double boiler. Add to the mixing bowl after the sugar and egg whites. Proceed as directed. SEE COLOR PLATE 7

MOCHA DACQUOISE

This is an indulgent bit of heaven. Make it for your chocolate-addicted friends. A small portion goes a long way. It is very rich. The light crispness of the meringue layers contrasts brilliantly with the creamy—no cream—pudding. This makes a four-layer pastry.

> 4 egg whites, at room temperature
> ⅓ cup sugar
> 1 teaspoon instant espresso powder
> 1 teaspoon unsweetened cocoa powder
> ½ recipe Chocolate Marsala Pudding (page 178)

Preheat the oven to 250°F with one rack in the top and another in the middle. Cover two 12-×-15-inch cookie sheets with a layer of parchment paper. Have ready a pastry bag with a ½-inch-diameter nozzle and set aside.

Place the egg whites in an electric mixer and start to beat slowly. Beat until frothy. Slowly add the sugar. Increase the speed to the fullest. Beat until the egg whites are very stiff. Fold in the espresso and cocoa powders.

Now move quickly or the mixture will not stay ideally firm: Spoon the stiff egg whites into the pastry bag. Pipe the meringue onto one half of one of the cookie sheets in a continuous spiral, starting from the center, until the round is about 6 inches in diameter. Make another meringue round on the same sheet and two more on the other sheet. Place both in the oven and bake for 45 minutes.

Turn off the oven and leave the meringues undisturbed for another 4½ hours. They should be crisp and dry. Remove the baking sheets from the oven and slide the meringues, still on their paper, onto a flat surface. The rounds will easily come off the parchment paper. Place one round flat and spread ⅓ cup pudding on top. Cover with another meringue round and repeat with the remaining pudding and rounds. Cut into wedges to serve.

SERVES 4 TO 6

CHOCOLATE MOUSSE

When I first started to cook, I looked at books—which was how I knew how to learn. For years I made the mousse from Dione Lucas's *Le Cordon Bleu Cook Book*. Now I have come up with my own simple and airy mousse that satisfies even my Viennese-born husband. It is still very rich, and a small amount is satisfying.

Use fresh organic eggs to avoid any health problems.

> 1 cup Chocolate Sauce (page 199), at room temperature
> 4 egg whites, at room temperature

Place the chocolate sauce in a medium bowl. Beat the egg whites until stiff peaks form. Gently fold a third of the egg whites into the chocolate sauce, then repeat with the remaining whites. Cover and refrigerate for 4 hours.

MAKES 3 CUPS

BLACKBERRY BAVARIAN CREAM

I have always made and enjoyed Bavarian creams. Usually they include whipped cream. I have been able to avoid it here to stunning effect.

Use fresh organic eggs to avoid any health problems.

6 cups fresh blackberries (about four 5½-ounce containers), plus extra for serving (see Note)

1 cup sugar

1 tablespooon unflavored gelatin (one and a half ¼-ounce packets)

1 cup coconut milk

3 eggs, separated

8 cups crushed ice or ice cubes

Combine the blackberries and sugar in a 3- to 4-quart saucepan. Cook over medium heat, stirring frequently, for 20 to 30 minutes, until the berries are very soft and mushy and have thrown off a generous amount of juice.

Remove from the heat and transfer to a large sieve with fine holes or a chinois set over a large mixing bowl. Using a wooden spoon, press the softened berries against the holes of the sieve to garner the crushed fruit and juices while removing the seeds and skins. You can help the process by periodically scraping the outside of the sieve with a rubber spatula. The cooked berries should produce 2 cups of juicy purée. Let the purée cool to room temperature.

In a microwave-safe glass measuring cup, sprinkle the gelatin over ½ cup cool water and let sit until the gelatin dissolves and the water becomes gelatinous, about 5 minutes. Cook in the microwave for 30 seconds, which will return the combination to liquid form. Let cool to room temperature.

In a 2- to 3-quart saucepan, whisk the coconut milk with the egg yolks until combined and smooth. Place the pan over medium-low heat and, stirring constantly, cook until somewhat thickened and the surface begins to appear more opaque, about 15 minutes. Remove from the heat but continue to stir until the soft custardlike mixture cools to body temperature, about 10 minutes.

In a separate and completely clean large mixing bowl, beat the egg whites, using an electric mixer with the whisk attachment. Beat at medium-low speed until the whites become frothy. Then increase the speed to high and whisk until the whites form stiff peaks but are not yet dry.

In an 8- to 10-quart metal mixing bowl, stir the blackberry purée with the gelatin mixture. Add the cooled custard and stir until smooth.

Fill a large glass or metal mixing bowl halfway with crushed ice or ice cubes and place the metal bowl containing the blackberry mixture on top of the ice. Continue filling the larger bowl with ice so that it comes up the sides of the smaller bowl and chills its surfaces. Immediately begin stirring the fruit mixture with a spatula, scraping the mixture from the sides of the cold bowl and also deep to the bottom of the bowl. It will gradually begin to thicken, becoming heavy. This step takes about 10 minutes.

Remove the bowl from the ice container and dump the egg whites all at once into the metal bowl. Using a rubber spatula, gently fold the egg whites into the fruit mixture, periodically turning the bowl so that all the egg whites are gradually incorporated into the fruit.

Chill a metal mold or bowl with crushed ice or ice cubes for at least 5 minutes, until icy cold. Discard the ice and pour the finished Bavarian cream mixture into the prepared mold. Smooth the top with the edge of a spatula. Cover and refrigerate until completely chilled, at least 2 hours.

To unmold, dip the mold into a bowl of hot tap water to loosen the sides. Cover with a serving plate and invert. Carefully remove the mold. Serve with extra blackberries.

SERVES 6

NOTE
Other berries can be used.

CHESTNUT DOUGHNUT HOLES

These are a delightful alternative to the gluten- and dairy-laden doughnut hole. SEE COLOR PLATE 11

Safflower oil for deep-frying
½ cup chestnut flour
¼ cup plus 1 tablespoon coconut milk
1 egg, separated

Pour oil 3 inches deep into a 4-quart saucepan. Place the pot over medium heat and bring the oil to 300°F. While the oil is heating, combine the flour, coconut milk, ¼ cup water, and the egg yolk in a medium bowl.

In a separate bowl, whisk the egg white or beat it in an electric mixer until it forms stiff peaks. Using a flexible spatula, fold the white into the chestnut batter, then set the bowl aside.

Constantly monitor the oil temperature to make sure that it stays at 300°F. To fry, drop 1 teaspoon at a time into the oil using a heat-resistant plastic spoon. Fry for 30 seconds, then flip over and fry for 20 seconds, until golden brown. Work carefully to avoid getting burned. Remove from the pot with a slotted spoon and place on a paper-towel-lined plate.

These can be tossed in sugar or served plain and enjoyed immediately or at room temperature.

MAKES 30 TO 35 PIECES

CHICKPEA BONBONS

These golden fried puffs can be prepared as a treat or as a savory snack—as in the variation—worthy of any cocktail party. The sweet preparation in the main recipe is a delight on its own or with fruit or sorbet. The hint of paprika in the savory preparation adds another dimension of flavor that makes these little bites an ideal companion to wine or beer.

Safflower oil for deep-frying
½ cup garbanzo bean (chickpea) flour
¼ cup plus 1 tablespoon coconut milk
1 egg, separated
2 tablespoons sugar, plus more for garnish

Pour oil 3 inches deep into a 4-quart saucepan. Place the pot over medium heat and heat the oil to 375°F.

While the oil is heating, combine the flour, coconut milk, ¼ cup water, the egg yolk, and the sugar in a medium bowl.

In a separate bowl, whisk the egg white until it forms stiff peaks. Using a spatula, fold the whites into the chickpea batter, then set the bowl aside. Continue to maintain the oil temperature at 375°F. For frying, scoop 1 teaspoon of the batter into a heat-resistant plastic spoon and drop the batter toward the sides of the pot, making sure to dip the spoon into the oil as you drop the batter. If these steps are ignored, the result will be flat discs rather than round bonbons. Fry for 30 seconds, then flip over and fry for 15 to 20 seconds, until golden brown. Remove from the pot with a slotted spoon and place on a paper-towel-lined plate.

Enjoy hot or warm. If need be, hold in a low oven, or allow to cool and fry again when ready to serve. Toss in sugar.

MAKES 30 TO 35 BONBONS

VARIATION

Spicy Chickpea Bonbons
Replace the sugar with 1 teaspoon salt and ½ teaspoon hot paprika. Proceed as directed. Toss with additional paprika.

CHESTNUT PANCAKE TORTE

This invention was inspired by an Austro-Hungarian classic made, of course, with ordinary flour. I think that the nutty sweetness of the chestnut flour is equally satisfying. The apricot filling between the layers is a classic, but it might be equally good with melted sweetened dark chocolate. This is a very rich torte, so a little goes a long way.

The pancakes are fragile. Handle with care.

APRICOT FILLING

1 vanilla bean (2 to 3 inches long)

½ cup dried apricots (about 3 ounces)

¼ cup sugar

2 tablespoons fresh lemon juice

2 teaspoons freshly grated lemon zest

PANCAKES

3 tablespoons safflower oil

½ cup chestnut flour

¼ cup teff flour

¾ cup coconut milk

2 eggs

MAKE THE FILLING: Break the vanilla bean into pieces into ½ cup water in a 2-cup glass measure. Cover tightly with plastic wrap and microwave for 30 seconds. Pierce the plastic with the tip of a sharp knife to release steam. Remove the cup from the oven and add the remaining filling ingredients.

Re-cover tightly with plastic wrap and microwave for 3½ minutes. Pierce the plastic with the tip of a sharp knife to release steam. Discard the vanilla bean. Using a spatula, scrape the contents of the cup into a food processor. Purée until smooth. Allow the mixture to cool.

MAKE THE PANCAKES: Whisk together 1 tablespoon of the oil and the remaining pancake ingredients in a medium bowl. Set aside.

Heat 1 teaspoon of the remaining oil in an 8- or 9-inch nonstick sauté pan over medium heat. Once the oil shimmers, reduce the heat to medium-low. Starting on the outer edge and working toward the middle, pour ¼ cup of batter into the pan, spreading it with a spatula to make a 6-inch crêpe. Cook for 2 minutes or until the edges are golden brown and the surface is completely dry, then carefully flip over with a spatula. Cook for 2 minutes, then slide onto a baking sheet. Repeat, using a teaspoon of oil for each pancake. Make sure to spread the pancakes out in a single layer on the baking sheet(s) so they overlap as little as possible while cooling. There will be six total.

Place one pancake on a serving plate. Spread evenly with 1 tablespoon of apricot purée, leaving a ½-inch border around the edge. Repeat with four more pancakes. Top the cake with the last pancake. Slice the cake with a sharp serrated knife.

MAKES ONE 6-LAYER CAKE; SERVES 4 TO 6

FROZEN DESSERTS

Well, here we get to the sorbets and some frozen desserts that resemble ice cream.

I heartily recommend the purchase of an electric sorbet machine with a removable bowl. Once it's on hand, it will actually be used. Keep a fair amount of Simple Syrup (page 184) on hand to make impulse desserts possible. The syrup needs to be refrigerated until cold before use.

Look at the sauces on pages 198–99 if you want to gussy up your dessert. The meringues (page 174), the Yum Yums (page 178), and the Bonbons (page 181) are possible accompaniments.

BANANA COCONUT ICE CREAM

This ice cream goes against all convention and actually tastes better after being in the freezer for a few days or weeks rather than when eaten fresh.

> 1 pound bananas, peeled and sliced (2 cups)
> ¼ cup coconut milk
> ¼ cup sugar
> ¼ cup fresh lime juice

Place the bananas, coconut milk, sugar, and lime juice in a food processor and blend until smooth. Using a spatula, scrape the mixture into an ice cream maker and churn for 35 minutes.

MAKES 1 QUART

MANGOSTEEN ICE CREAM

This may be one of the world's most expensive desserts. It is well worth it when the fruit is in season—usually in our spring. The fruit has a tough skin that needs to be cut to be peeled away. Inside the fruit will be white and look much like lychees. It has numerous pits.

> 2½ pounds fresh mangosteens, peeled, pitted, and cut into chunks (about 2 cups)
> ¼ cup coconut milk
> ¼ cup sugar

Place the mangosteen chunks, coconut milk, and sugar in a food processor and blend until smooth. Using a spatula, scrape the mixture into an ice cream maker and churn for 35 to 40 minutes.

MAKES 1 PINT

SORBETS

I have gotten to the point at which I am almost tempted to swear at very decent and kind wait staff in restaurants who are aware of my dietary peculiarities and tell me sweetly that there are lovely sorbets and fresh fruit. That is the response in almost every restaurant. The fact that I can also have these at home does not make the restaurant versions more appealing.

I do in fact make sorbets—very good ones, because fresh is better. I have gone so far as to buy excellent sorbet machines that self-chill. I put the sorbet into one as we sit down to eat, and it is finished in time to be dessert. I include some of my favorites here. The basic rule is simple: one part—say 4 cups—of puréed fruit to an equal amount of simple syrup. Often, I add some lemon juice, particularly when using purée put up and jarred in the summer. The juice freshens up the taste.

If the sorbet isn't perfectly smooth, call it "granite" and enjoy.

THREE WAYS TO FREEZE SORBETS

USING AN ICE CREAM MAKER

If the sorbet mixture has been heated, refrigerate it, then pour it into the ice cream maker and follow the manufacturer's directions.

USING ICE CUBE TRAYS

Pour the base into old-fashioned ice cube trays—you have them in a closet somewhere. Freeze overnight or until solid and then, right before serving, purée in a blender or food processor until fluffy.

USING FREEZER CONTAINERS

No ice cube trays? Put the mixture into freezer containers that hold about a pint. From time to time, stir with a fork and, as the sorbet hardens, scrape with the fork and stir in.

WHITE PEACH PURÉE

This purée can be the base for a refreshing summer sorbet. I use many things out of the garden or in plentiful, cheap supply from the farmers' market to make sorbets (pages 185–87). I often freeze them to have on hand to make it easy.

1½ pounds peaches, pitted and cut up, unpeeled
½ cup sugar

Stir the peaches and sugar together in a medium saucepan. Bring to a boil over medium heat. Reduce to simmer. Cook, stirring from time to time, until the peaches are almost mush, about 1 hour. Put through the fine disc of a food mill.

MAKES ENOUGH TO MAKE 6 PINTS SORBET

SIMPLE SYRUP

Simple syrup is often used to sweeten cold drinks—alcoholic and non—as the sugar is already dissolved. It is also used to make sorbet. It sweetens the dish but also keeps it from degenerating into large crystals.

The simple syrup given here is a one-to-one syrup, meaning one part water to one part sugar. Sometimes a heavier syrup made with two parts sugar to one part water is desired, or, conversely, a lighter one made with one part sugar to two parts water.

Boiling the syrup not only dissolves the sugar but also stabilizes the mixture.

2 cups sugar

Combine the sugar with 2 cups water in a small saucepan. Over high heat, bring to a boil. Reduce the heat to a simmer until the sugar is dissolved, about 5 minutes.

MAKES 3 CUPS

LEMON SORBET

This is light, fresh, and delicious, but it doesn't follow the general rules for sorbet. Think of it as smoothly frozen lemonade. It is a very pale yellow—almost white. A sprig of mint would not be amiss. I prefer Meyer lemons.

> **1 cup sugar**
>
> **1 cup plus 2 tablespoons fresh lemon juice (from 6 to 8 lemons)**

Bring the sugar and 3 cups water to a boil in a medium saucepan. Reduce the heat and simmer until all the sugar is dissolved, about 5 minutes. Refrigerate until cold. Stir in the lemon juice and pour into a sorbet machine or use one of the methods opposite.

MAKES 4 CUPS

PINEAPPLE SORBET

This is one of my favorites. It comes out almost white and fluffy. Save the unused parts of a large pineapple for another day, or cut in chunks to go with sorbet.

> **1 pineapple (3½ to 4 pounds), peeled, cored, and cut into 2-inch chunks (5 to 6 cups)**
>
> **3 cups Simple Syrup (opposite)**
>
> **Fresh lemon juice to taste**

Place the pineapple chunks in a food processor and process until the purée is smooth and has no visible chunks. Add the simple syrup and lemon juice and mix until combined. Finish in a sorbet machine, or use one of the methods opposite.

MAKES 1 QUART

PINEAPPLE BASICS

CLEANING

Slice off the top and bottom of the pineapple. Discard. Stand the pineapple flat on the work surface. Cut down the sides with a knife until all the peel is removed.

Trim away the "eyes" with the tip of a vegetable peeler or by cutting diagonal grooves along the outside of the pineapple and eliminating multiple eyes at once. Quarter the pineapple.

Lay each quarter flat and lengthwise on the work surface. Positioning the knife at an angle, cut out the core of the pineapple and set aside. Cut the pineapple quarters into ½-inch slices. Enjoy immediately or use as desired. A 4-pound pineapple makes about 6 cups.

PURÉEING

Place 6 cups of pineapple slices in a food processor and purée until smooth.

MAKES 4 CUPS PURÉE

NOTES

One pound of unprocessed (raw, unpeeled, not trimmed of scrap) pineapple makes roughly 1 cup purée, so a 3-pound pineapple will produce 3 cups purée, a 4-pound pineapple will produce 4 cups purée, and so on.

The core of the pineapple can be sliced and enjoyed as a snack or cut into slender skewers about ¼ inch thick and 5 to 7 inches long (depending on how long the pineapple was). The skewers make for a beautiful presentation but are not nearly as tasty after they have been exposed to heat.

CHOCOLATE SORBET

Years ago, I included a chocolate sorbet with rum in *The Four Seasons Cookbook*. Here I have substituted Triple Sec for a slight jolt of orange. The sorbet is so rich that I fear no one believes there is no cream.

> **6 ounces unsweetened chocolate (about 70% cacao)**
> **1 cup sugar**
> **3 tablespoons Triple Sec**
> **½ teaspoon vanilla extract**

Chop the chocolate into very small pieces, either in a food processor or with a knife. In a saucepan, bring the chocolate, 2 cups water, and the sugar to a boil over medium heat, stirring constantly. Reduce the heat to low and cook for about 8 minutes, stirring all the while, or until the mixture is completely smooth. Let cool to room temperature and add the Triple Sec and vanilla.

Finish in a sorbet machine or use one of the methods on page 184.

MAKES 2½ CUPS

CRANBERRY SORBET

The one time of the year that many people cook and also think of cranberries is Thanksgiving. While it is better to cook and think of cranberries at least once annually, it is truly a shame that we don't cook cranberries more often. This sensational sorbet can be a refreshing and beautiful end to any midwinter meal. It looks particularly nice when served in Champagne glasses. I serve it with a few cookies and am happy.

> **2 juice oranges**
> **One 12-ounce bag cranberries (about 3½ cups)**
> **2 cups Simple Syrup (page 184)**

Using a vegetable peeler, remove six 2-inch strips of zest from the oranges. Juice the oranges to get ½ cup juice.

Combine the cranberries, orange juice, zest, and ¼ cup of the syrup in a medium saucepan. Bring to a boil, reduce the heat, and simmer over very low heat for 40 minutes or until the cranberries have almost completely liquefied. Put the mixture through a food mill fitted with the fine-hole disc. Stir in the remaining 1¾ cups syrup and 1 cup water. Chill, covered, until cold, about 2 hours. The recipe can be done ahead up to this point.

Finish in a sorbet machine or use one of the methods on page 184.

MAKES 5½ CUPS

PAPAYA SORBET

The reddish Hawaiian papayas now on the market make this sorbet particularly attractive.

2 medium papayas, peeled, seeded, and cut into chunks

1 cup Simple Syrup (page 184)

Juice of 3 limes

Purée the papaya in a food processor until smooth. There should be about 1½ cups purée. Add the syrup and lime juice.

Finish in a sorbet machine or use one of the methods on page 184.

MAKES ABOUT 2 CUPS

MANGOSTEEN SORBET

This is a lot lighter and a lot cheaper and easier than the Mangosteen Ice Cream (page 183). It is perfect for lunch on a hot summer's day. The whole kitchen will smell delightfully of the juice as it reduces.

Those who want a little extra jazz can pour a little potato vodka over each portion. It is even possible to make this into a drink by using a Champagne glass and more vodka or Champagne.

Four 12-ounce cans mangosteen juice

Pour all the juice into a medium saucepan over low heat. Reduce by half, which will take about 30 minutes. Pour the reduced juice into an ice cream maker and process for about 35 minutes.

Finish in a sorbet machine or use one of the methods on page 184.

MAKES 4 CUPS

SAUCES

I am not French and therefore do not have a tendency to top or toss each dish with a sauce; but sauces certainly have their uses. It has taken some work to develop a group of sauces that meet my "intolerant" needs. Several come from the classic repertoire, and others are modest inventions.

Use seasonings as one would any other spice in the kitchen. Taste and invent.

THE MAYONNAISES

Mayonnaise is a splendid French invention named after a general. The technique is very adaptable (see Chocolate Marsala Pudding, page 178).

BASIC MAYONNAISE

This is the ultimate adaptable sauce. Thin it out with a tablespoon or so of water and heat slightly for a reasonable hollandaise sauce substitute. Add fresh herbs and chopped cooked spinach for a green sauce. Add capers, chopped onion, chopped parsley, and chopped gherkins for tartar sauce. Add Tomato Purée (page 208) for a pretty, cold sauce for fish. Add some grainy mustard or horseradish to make a spread for cold loin of pork (see page 121).

The mayonnaise can also be made in a blender (add the oil more quickly) or with a whisk (add the oil more slowly). Save the egg whites for meringues (see page 174).

> 3 egg yolks, at room temperature
> 1½ tablespoons fresh lemon juice
> 1½ teaspoons kosher salt
> Freshly ground white pepper
> 1 teaspoon dry mustard
> 1 cup safflower oil
> 1 cup good virgin olive oil

Place the egg yolks in a food processor and process for 90 seconds. Stop the machine and add the lemon juice, salt, pepper, and mustard. Process with 2 short pulses to mix.

Pour the oils into a measuring cup. Beginning very slowly but steadily, pour the oil into the running food processor. When about a third of the oil has been added, increase the rate at which you're adding oil slightly and continue adding it until it has all been absorbed. Refrigerate in a closed jar. It will keep for a good week.

MAKES 2 CUPS

MY FAVORITE MAYO

Super as a topping on baked potatoes and just as good on firm cooked vegetables or with artichokes.

> 2 egg yolks
> ¼ cup Simple Superior Sauce (page 197)
> 1 cup olive oil

Place the yolks in a blender. Pour in the sauce and whir for 30 seconds. Gradually, with the machine running, pour in the olive oil. This mayo will keep for a week.

MAKES 1½ CUPS

CURRY MAYONNAISE

This goes particularly well with fish or fresh red bell pepper.

> 1 cup mayonnaise (homemade [above or left], or store-bought)
> 1 tablespoon plus 1 teaspoon Curry Vinaigrette (page 196)

Whisk the mayonnaise and vinaigrette together in a small bowl until well combined. Serve immediately or cover and refrigerate for up to a week.

MAKES 1 CUP

ROE SAUCE

Any mayo requires good olive oil, salt, and some acid—lemon, vinegar, lime. It also requires eggs. The usual ones are hen eggs, although fish eggs are used here. All the ingredients need to be at room temperature and good quality.

My first mayonnaise experiment—very good too—was in Aspen at the house of a fabulous fisher. She had returned from a high-mountain trip, where it was legal to keep your trout catch. I volunteered to be the cook. First I had to clean the fish. As I cleaned, I noted that some of the fish were ladies with egg sacs. What to do? I made a sauce with the eggs. It was sensational. Since then, I have gone on to using other fish roes when available. I wouldn't use beluga or other glamorous roes, but there are many that are good and that work.

When buying fish, ask the monger to save the roe for you. Incidentally, striped bass roe can be poached and served as you would the most elegant of quenelles. Bottled roe can also be used. Experiment; have fun.

3 ounces fish roe, such as shad roe

½ cup mild but good olive oil

¼ teaspoon salt

Juice of ½ lemon

Place the roe in a blender and blend to break it up some. While the blender is running, slowly pour in the oil until the mixture is a thick mayonnaise consistency. Stir in the salt and lemon juice. Serve this sauce with cod or chicken.

MAKES ⅔ CUP

AÏOLI

Aïoli is a garlicky mayonnaise from southern France. In this recipe, I add a few drops of hot pepper sauce, which is definitely not classic. If you need aïoli for vegetables, just omit the hot sauce.

2 large eggs

1 tablespoon plus 1 teaspoon fresh lemon juice

12 drops hot red pepper sauce, such as Tabasco

2 teaspoons kosher salt

¼ teaspoon freshly ground black pepper

½ cup light olive oil

6 to 8 cloves garlic, to taste, smashed and peeled

Put the eggs, lemon juice, hot pepper sauce, salt, and pepper into a food processor. Process until well blended. With the machine running, pour in the oil in a steady stream until it is incorporated and the mayonnaise is smooth. Add the garlic. Process until smooth. The mayonnaise is now an aïoli. It will keep for at least a week.

MAKES 1 CUP

OTHER SAUCES

Many dishes are enhanced by a sauce, whether savory or sweet. Sauces are a wonderful playground for the inventive cook, and I myself have had a great deal of fun developing these.

SWEET PEA MUSH SAUCE

One weekend I had a vegan over for dinner. I decided on Mushroom Risotto (page 43) and, as a first course, some Spanish white asparagus with a classic hollandaise sauce. But then it occurred to me: no egg yolks, no anchovies . . . no sauce. That was when scarcity hit. I rummaged in the cabinets and didn't even have any canned chickpeas to make my new Basic Best Sauce (see page 53).

I did have a can of tiny little peas for which I have a low-taste weakness. I thought "Why not?" If chickpeas can work as a thickener or sauce, why not another starch? And so, scarcity inspired this new recipe, which is so delicious it could even replace guacamole.

> One 14-ounce can petite sweet peas, drained
> 2 cloves garlic, smashed, peeled, and cut into chunks
> ¼ cup olive oil
> Juice of ½ Meyer lemon, or a little more of a regular lemon
> Kosher salt

Put the peas in a food processor and process until puréed. Add the garlic, olive oil, and lemon juice, then process until the whole mixture is smooth. Season with salt to taste.

Allow the sauce to sit for an hour to mellow the flavors before serving. It is best used that day.

MAKES 1½ CUPS

TOMATO AND LOVAGE SAUCE

Lovage tastes like a blend of celery, parsley, and tarragon, with a hint of curry. The most popular herb in ancient Roman times, it has virtually disappeared from contemporary recipes, which is a shame. Cooked, it adds robust backbone to stews and sauces. Small raw leaves can be added whole into salads or cooked dishes. To avoid stringiness, stems should not be used, and larger leaves should be cut across like sorrel.

Difficult to find even in farmers' markets, lovage is easy to grow outdoors, especially if grown by buying a plant or taking a rooted clump from a friend's plant. Just be careful where you put it; lovage quickly reaches gargantuan proportions, about 6 feet high and 5 feet wide. Lovage likes full sun, too, and produces sprays of 3- to 5-inch leaves on celerylike plants.

This sauce is good on gluten-free pasta, in stews, and with poached chicken or fish.

> 1 tablespoon olive oil
> 1 small onion, cut into ¼-inch dice (about ¾ cup)
> 4 medium cremini mushrooms, trimmed, cut in half, and then cut lengthwise into ¼-inch-thick slices
> 2 medium cloves garlic, smashed, peeled, and minced
> 3 medium tomatoes, cut into ¼-inch dice (2 cups)
> ¼ cup lovage leaves, cut across into thin strips
> Kosher salt
> Freshly ground black pepper

Heat the oil in a medium-large skillet over medium heat. Add the onion and stir to coat in the oil. Cook, stirring occasionally, for 2 minutes. Add the mushrooms and garlic. Cook, stirring occasionally, for 3 minutes. Add the tomatoes and cook for 5 minutes or until the tomatoes have collapsed. Stir in the lovage and cook for 2 minutes more. Roughly purée in a food processor. Season with salt and pepper to taste.

MAKES 3 CUPS

TOMATO SAUCE CASALINGA (HOME STYLE)

This is my everyday tomato sauce. I suggest making the largest amount possible and keeping it on hand not only for a quick, comforting, and filling bowl of gluten-free pasta but also to have with almost any kind of simply cooked chicken, fish, or meat (I wouldn't put it on beef). Keep some in the freezer and some in the refrigerator.

As a pasta sauce, I like it with gluten-free spaghettini. If fresh basil is available, toss some in when mixing the pasta with the sauce. While these quantities look huge, I normally make the sauce and then use it as needed.

This sauce is very low in calories, so add as much as you'd like to any dish. Because it's made in the microwave, there's less chance of burning.

1 tablespoon olive oil

4 garlic cloves, smashed, peeled, and finely chopped

1 small onion (2 ounces), finely chopped
(about ½ cup)

1 small carrot, peeled and finely chopped
(about ¼ cup)

1 small stalk celery, peeled and finely chopped
(about ¼ cup)

2 medium white mushrooms, trimmed and
thinly sliced (about ¾ cup)

One 35-ounce can Italian plum tomatoes,
packed in juice

½ teaspoon dried oregano

½ teaspoon dried basil

1 tablespoon fresh lemon juice

1 teaspoon kosher salt

Pinch freshly ground black pepper

Combine the olive oil and two of the garlic cloves in the center of a 2½-quart soufflé dish or casserole. Cook, uncovered, in the microwave, on high for 2 minutes. Add the onion, carrot, celery, and mushrooms and cook, uncovered, for 3 minutes.

Stir in the tomatoes and their liquid, the oregano, the basil, and the remaining garlic. Cook, uncovered, for 7 minutes, stirring twice. Remove from the oven and let stand until cool.

Add the lemon juice, salt, and pepper. Working in batches, process the sauce in a blender at low speed until smooth. Refrigerate, covered, for up to 7 days or freeze for up to 6 months.

MAKES 4½ CUPS

SPRING VEGETABLE TOMATO SAUCE WITH MINT

This sauce on pasta can be a fresh way to start a meal or be one. Choose gluten-free penne.

⅜ cup olive oil

¼ pound mushrooms (4 or 5 medium), trimmed and cut into ¼-inch slices (about 1¾ cups)

1 small onion, finely chopped (about ⅓ cup)

1 cup (¾ pound) shelled peas

1½ cups Tomato Purée (homemade, page 208, or store-bought)

½ cup white wine

¼ cup minced mint leaves (about ½ cup packed whole leaves)

2 teaspoons kosher salt

Pour 2 tablespoons of the oil into a 10-inch skillet over high heat. When the oil shimmers, add the mushrooms. Cook until golden brown, 3 to 4 minutes. Add the onion and cook until it begins to wilt. Stir in the peas and cook for 1 minute.

Turn the heat down so the mixture is just bubbling. Add the tomato purée and cook for 3 to 4 minutes more. Pour in the remaining olive oil and cook the sauce for 3 minutes more or until the peas are nearly done. Stir in the wine and then the mint. Bring to a boil, then reduce the heat to simmer. Season with the salt.

MAKES 2½ CUPS, ENOUGH FOR 6 SERVINGS OF PASTA

GREEN VELVET CILANTRO SAUCE

I devised this sauce for the Salmon Shiitake Kebabs on page 80. It is such a beautiful color and the flavor is so delicious that I have now used it on other things. A tablespoon can be mixed into each chopped hard-boiled egg for a salad. It is yummy with any simple fish and even poached chicken. And it works well on pasta.

1 piece ginger (about 2 ounces), peeled and chopped

1 bunch cilantro (4 to 5 ounces), stemmed (about ½ cup tightly packed leaves)

2 cloves garlic, smashed, peeled, and coarsely chopped

1 cup coconut milk

2 tablespoons gluten-free soy sauce

½ teaspoon ground turmeric

1 tablespoon fresh lime juice

Place all the ingredients in a blender and process until smooth.

MAKES 1½ CUPS

GIBLET GRAVY

Giblet gravy is easy if time consuming, and the basic principle is the same no matter what the size of the bird. The measurements here are for a 15-pound turkey. It's not pan gravy; make it up to 2 days ahead.

> Wing tips, giblets (heart and gizzards), and neck from a 15-pound turkey or 2 chickens
>
> 6 garlic cloves, smashed and peeled
>
> 3½ cups chicken stock (any of the homemade stocks, pages 203–4, or sterile-pack)
>
> 1 tablespoon chopped fresh herbs (optional)
>
> Kosher salt
>
> Freshly ground black pepper

Put the wing tips, giblets, neck, garlic, and stock in the smallest pan that will hold the ingredients comfortably. Cover and bring to a boil. Reduce the heat to simmer, skim, and cook, uncovered, for 2 hours or until the giblets are easily pierced with the point of a knife. Add 1 cup water each time the liquid has reduced by half. Do not start with more liquid or stock, or the gravy will not be a rich, dark color. Skim occasionally. Remove the giblets, allowing them to cool.

Continue to cook the stock for 2 hours, until the neck bones fall apart. Add water as needed. For the last 20 minutes, let cook without adding any more water. Cut the heart and gizzards into thin slices or small cubes and reserve. Strain the stock. Skim off any remaining fat. Just before serving, add the giblets and, if you wish, some fresh herbs. Pick the meat from the neck and add. Heat until warm throughout. Add the deglazing liquid from the roasted bird if available. Season with salt and pepper to taste.

MAKES 2½ CUPS

BASIC VINAIGRETTE

Use this vinaigrette to dress a salad, coat vegetables, or as a marinade.

> ¼ cup fresh lemon juice
>
> 1 cup olive oil
>
> 2 teaspoons kosher salt

Whisk all the ingredients together in a small bowl.

MAKES 1¼ CUPS

ENRICHED VINAIGRETTE

This vinaigrette is another classic often used on salads with fish, meat, or eggs in them. I use it as an alternate on the Herb-Simmered Leg of Lamb (page 134).

> 10 sprigs flat-leaf parsley, stemmed and coarsely chopped
>
> 1 tablespoon plus 1 teaspoon anchovy paste
>
> 1 tablespoon Dijon mustard
>
> 1 teaspoon kosher salt
>
> 1 teaspoon freshly ground black pepper
>
> ½ cup red wine vinegar
>
> 1 cup olive oil
>
> ¼ cup drained capers, coarsely chopped
>
> 2 hard-boiled eggs, finely chopped

In a food processor, pulse the parsley, anchovy paste, mustard, salt, pepper, and vinegar to combine. With the machine running, slowly pour in the oil. Scrape into a small bowl and stir in the capers and eggs.

MAKES 3 CUPS

CURRY VINAIGRETTE

This is divine on cold fish. Use it also to dress a salad, coat vegetables, or as a marinade. Make it ahead as it thickens up over time.

> 2 tablespoons curry powder
> ½ cup olive oil
> ½ cup fresh lime juice
> 2½ teaspoons kosher salt

Combine the curry powder and olive oil in a small pot over low heat. Bring to a simmer and heat for 1 minute. Whisk in the lime juice and salt. Using a spatula, scrape the contents into a bowl. Allow to cool.

MAKES 1 GENEROUS CUP

SARDINE SAUCE

This is the basic sauce for Herb-Simmered Leg of Lamb (page 134).

> 3 large eggs
> 3 cups olive oil
> Six 3.75-ounce cans oil-packed sardines, drained, boned if need be, and lightly crushed
> 5 tablespoons green peppercorns packed in brine, drained and rinsed
> 3 tablespoons tarragon vinegar
> 1½ teaspoons kosher salt

In a food processor, pulse the eggs until slightly foamy, about 5 times. With the machine running, pour the oil through the feed tube a few drops at a time. When about a cup has been added and the sauce starts to thicken, pour a little faster, in a slow, steady stream, until the oil has been incorporated.

Add the sardines and 2 tablespoons of the peppercorns. Pulse to combine, about 10 times. Add the vinegar and salt and pulse to combine.

Scrape the sauce into a medium bowl and stir in the remaining peppercorns.

MAKES 6 CUPS

SIMPLE SUPERIOR SAUCE FOR STEAMED, POACHED, OR BOILED FOODS

Yes, it sounds pretentious, but this sauce does live up to the title's promise. I originally made it for poached leeks and have gone on to use it on steamed Belgian endive, microwave-cooked or boiled cauliflower, jarred white asparagus, microwave-cooked asparagus, as well as steamed chicken and white-fleshed fish, steamed and roasted. I have yet to try it on pork or veal; but as I keep extra in the refrigerator, I am sure the day will come.

Tins of anchovies that have been sitting overly long in the cupboard are fine because firm anchovies are not needed. It would even be possible to substitute anchovy paste from a tube—about a tablespoon. If using paste or if the olive oil in the tin is scanty, add an extra tablespoon of olive oil for each batch of the recipe. If the food to be sauced hasn't been poached, simply substitute chicken or fish stock for the cooking liquid. If doubling the recipe—it keeps well in the refrigerator—use only a cup of the liquid and then stir it into the finished sauce.

> One 2-ounce tin oil-packed flat anchovies
> 1 cup chicken stock (any of the homemade stocks, pages 203–4, or sterile-pack) or fish stock (page 205)
> 2 tablespoons drained capers
> 1 tablespoon balsamic vinegar
> 1 tablespoon olive oil (if the anchovies have little oil)

Put all the ingredients in a blender and process until smooth. Allow the sauce to sit and mellow for at least 30 minutes before using it.

MAKES 1½ CUPS

VARIATIONS

Endive Sauce for Four

Use ½ pound Belgian endives, trimmed. Place in the basket of a steamer. Place over 2 cups of stock. Cover. Bring to a boil. Reduce to a simmer and cook for about 20 minutes or until a knife slips easily into the endives. Make the sauce using endive stock. Serve the endives with sauce on the side and a spoon for eating. Serves about four.

Leek Sauce

Clean about 2 pounds of leeks, Cut off the root ends and cut leeks to have about 6 inches of white. Put in a pan large enough to hold them in a single layer. Cover with chicken stock, 1 quart or more. Cover. Bring to a boil and reduce to a simmer. Cook about 20 minutes or until the tip of a knife slides in easily. Make the sauce using the leek stock. Serve hot or cold with sauce.

APPLESAUCE

Quarter 5 pounds of smallish, firm apples—windfalls are fine. Put in a large pot with 4 cups water and 1 cup sugar. Bring to a boil. Lower the heat and cook until the apples are very soft. Put through the medium disc of a food mill to get about 8 cups of sauce. Let cool and stir in the juice of 2 lemons. Will keep refrigerated for up to 1 month.

RHUBARB CHUTNEY

One of the cheering sights of spring is rhubarb, whether as big-leafed plants in the garden or as strong red stalks in the market. Cooks usually think of rhubarb in terms of sweet dishes like compote, pie, or jam, often mixed with strawberries. But it is a wonderful addition to the savory pantry as well.

This chutney goes particularly well with duck, pork, and other rich meats. The red of the rhubarb is reinforced by the fresh red radishes.

> 2 tablespoons plus 2 teaspoons safflower oil
>
> 4 medium shallots, cut into ¼-inch dice
>
> ⅓ cup diced peeled ginger
>
> 2 tablespoons curry powder
>
> 1 cup dark brown sugar
>
> 2¼ pounds rhubarb stalks, trimmed and cut diagonally into ½-inch pieces
>
> 15 medium red radishes, halved and cut across into thin slices

In a medium saucepan, heat the oil over medium heat. Stir in the shallots, ginger, and curry powder. Cook, stirring, for about 6 minutes or until the shallots are limp.

Stir in the brown sugar, rhubarb, and radishes. Cover the pot and raise the heat to medium-high. Cook, stirring occasionally, for 8 minutes or until the rhubarb is tender but not mushy.

If canned or frozen, this will keep indefinitely; refrigerated, it will keep for up to 1 month.

MAKES ABOUT 5 CUPS

RASPBERRY SAUCE

Fresh raspberries transform into a wonderful brightly colored sauce that pairs with anything chocolate and elevates Waffles (page 16) to an eye-catching dessert. SEE COLOR PLATE 6

> 2 half-pints raspberries (about ¾ pound)
> 2 tablespoons sugar
> 1 teaspoon fresh lemon juice (optional)

Place the berries in a food processor and process until smooth. Strain the mixture through a fine sieve into a small saucepan. Place the saucepan over medium heat, add the sugar, and stir until dissolved. Remove from the heat and allow to cool. If you need more acid, add the lemon juice.

MAKES ¾ CUP

VERY SPECIAL WILD STRAWBERRY SAUCE

Wild strawberries set their own schedule, have a season of only a few days, and do not keep well. When I have any, I make this sauce. The recipe is for a very small quantity but can easily be multiplied. One of the advantages is that the berries do not need to be hulled, which is a tiresome chore. Use to drizzle on Lemon Sorbet (page 185), to perk up domestic strawberries, or just eat greedily off a spoon.

> ¼ pound wild strawberries (about 1¾ cups)
> ½ cup sugar

Cook the strawberries and sugar in a stainless-steel pot until the sugar is dissolved and the berries are very soft. Put through a chinois or other very fine sieve. Enjoy.

MAKES ⅓ CUP

CHOCOLATE SAUCE

Chocolate sauce can turn an ordinary breakfast waffle (page 16) into a scrumptious dessert. This recipe also can be doubled or halved easily. Want a thicker sauce for coating, dipping, or fondue? Reduce the coconut milk by half. Be sure to use a high-quality dark chocolate that is about 70 percent cacao and milk-free. This also makes a base for Chocolate Mousse (page 179).

> 1½ cups coconut milk
> 7 ounces dark chocolate (about 70% cacao), broken into little pieces
> 1 teaspoon vanilla extract
> 2 tablespoons sugar

Place the coconut milk in a small saucepan over very low heat. Add the chocolate pieces and stir occasionally until completely melted. Pour in the vanilla and sugar and mix well.

MAKES 2 CUPS

ZABAGLIONE

This is an Italian classic usually served over sliced strawberries. It can be used as a lactose-free topping for desserts.

> 3 egg yolks
> ¼ cup gluten-free confectioners' sugar
> ⅓ cup Marsala

Combine the yolks and sugar in a blender and process for 1 to 2 minutes or until they increase in volume and turn pale yellow. Pour the mixture and the Marsala into a double boiler over medium heat. Whisk constantly until the mixture has nearly doubled in volume and become a light, airy beige sauce. This will take 5 to 10 minutes, depending on how hot your stove is and how much air you whisk into the mixture.

MAKES ¾ CUP

BASIC RECIPES

Here are seasoning powders, "preserved" lemons, purées, stocks, and bases. These recipes can be used with various foods in the book. Some can be made ahead in the amount that is preferred and kept in sealed containers either at room temperature, refrigerated, or frozen.

SEASONINGS

Sometimes we want a zap of flavor. These prepared ingredients can be kept on hand for a cook's craving.

BARBARA'S FIVE-SPICE POWDER

This is my own special seasoning blend that can be used in or on many things. It keeps well in a tightly closed container in the refrigerator, so it is worth multiplying. It is used in Spicy Kisses (page 29) and Simplest Lunch (page 68).

> ½ teaspoon ground star anise (1 or 2 whole star anise; see Note)
>
> 1 teaspoon ground turmeric
>
> ⅓ teaspoon kosher salt
>
> ½ teaspoon ground cumin
>
> ¼ teaspoon ground allspice
>
> ⅛ teaspoon cayenne pepper

Place the star anise in a mini food processor (or coffee grinder) and pulse until pulverized. Pour the powder into a mesh strainer over a small metal bowl to get rid of any remaining chunks. Add the other ingredients and mix well.

MAKES 1 TABLESPOON

NOTE

Eight to 10 whole star anise (¼ ounce) will make 1 generous tablespoon of ground star anise.

LEMON ZESTY SPICE MIX

Another spice mix I whipped up and like to keep on hand. Think fish and chicken as well as desserts. Multiply and store in a plastic container in the refrigerator.

> ½ teaspoon kosher salt
>
> ½ teaspoon anise seeds
>
> 6 whole black peppercorns
>
> Two 3-inch strips lemon zest

Place all the ingredients in a mini food processor or coffee grinder and pulse until the mixture resembles coarse sand.

MAKES 1 GENEROUS TEASPOON

"PRESERVED" LEMONS

This is cheating; but I think that it is a triumph. It permits me to make Moroccan dishes without having had the forethought to make real preserved lemons. The recipe can easily be multiplied if you like to cook Moroccan food often. The entire lemon is edible and silky. If you want to make the genuine article, read Paula Wolfert. This version will get closer to her kind by keeping in the refrigerator for about a month. Watch out for seasonings when using the lemons, which are very salty.

> 1 cup kosher salt
>
> 2 lemons, washed, trimmed of ends, each cut lengthwise into 6 wedges, seeds removed
>
> 2 tablespoons fresh lemon juice

Place the salt and 1 cup water in a medium saucepan over high heat (the liquid will be oversaturated, and the salt will eventually precipitate). Add the lemons, skin side down, and simmer for 30 minutes. Drain the lemons; rinse once, place in a container covered with the lemon juice, and allow to cool.

MAKES 12 WEDGES

PURÉES, STOCKS, AND BASES

Foods can of course be cooked or eaten raw on their own. However, using stock or a homemade base in the cooking gives extra flavor.

BASIC CHICKEN STOCK

Chicken stock is not difficult to make from scratch. I usually start it after I roast a chicken, using the carcass, innards, and any bones that I can snatch back from people's plates. Don't worry; they will be boiled. The remnants of each 5-pound chicken will make about a quart of stock.

I cook these stocks for a long time so as to extract the silky gelatin from the bones.

Freeze in pint containers for ease of use. Defrost in the microwave for about 5 minutes. A quart will defrost in about 9 minutes.

> **5 pounds chicken backs and necks, roasted carcasses, or other bones**

TO START THE STOCK ON TOP OF THE STOVE: In a tall, narrow stockpot, bring the bones and 3 quarts water to a boil. Skim the fat. Lower the heat and simmer gently, so bubbles are barely breaking the surface of the liquid, for at least 4 hours and up to 12; add water as needed to keep the bones covered. Skim as necessary to remove as much fat as possible.

TO START THE STOCK IN THE OVEN: Place a rack on the lowest level of the oven (remove any other racks) and heat the oven to 250°F.

In a tall, narrow stockpot on the stovetop, bring the bones and 3 quarts water to a boil. Skim the fat. Place in the oven for 4 hours; add water if needed. Remove and skim the fat. Return to the oven for at least 5 hours and up to 8.

TO START THE STOCK IN A SLOW COOKER: Start with 2½ pounds bones and 6 cups water for a 4-quart cooker. Place the bones in the slow cooker and pour the water over them. Cover and turn the heat to low. Cook for 11 to 12 hours.

TO FINISH USING ANY METHOD: The bones will be falling apart when the stock is done. Strain the stock through a fine-mesh sieve. Skim the fat and cool to room temperature. Refrigerate for 3 hours.

Remove the fat from the top of the stock and the sediment from the bottom. Use immediately, refrigerate for up to 3 days, or freeze.

MAKES 10 CUPS ON TOP OF THE STOVE, 8 CUPS IN THE OVEN, 6 CUPS IN THE SLOW COOKER

EXTRA-RICH CHICKEN STOCK

This recipe produces a very strong, rich, and delicious gelatinous stock. Don't use it for most cold soups, as they will turn solid; but it is perfect for aspics or gelled soups.

6 pounds chicken backs and necks

In a tall, narrow stockpot, bring the bones and 4 quarts plus 1 cup water to a boil. Skim the fat. Lower the heat and simmer gently, so the bubbles are barely breaking on the surface, for 12 hours, skimming the fat as necessary. Partially covering the pot with a lid will mean less evaporation.

Strain through a fine-mesh sieve. Skim the fat. Cool to room temperature. Refrigerate for 3 hours.

Remove the solidified fat from the top of the stock and the sediment (flip the gelled stock out of the container and scrape off the layer of sediment that has settled on the bottom). Use immediately, refrigerate for up to 3 days, or freeze.

MAKES 8 CUPS

FAKE CHICKEN STOCK

This is not a "real" stock because it's not made with bones from scratch. The added gelatin makes up for more bones. It's quicker than the other homemade stocks. When I have only a little time, however, it can enrich a commercially bought sterile-pack chicken stock, really enhancing it.

6 cups sterile-pack chicken broth or 6 cups water with the appropriate number of stock cubes

1 pound chicken bones, backs, necks, or wings or a combination

1 large yellow onion, skin on, quartered

Two ¼-ounce packets gelatin (14 to 15 grams total weight)

In a medium saucepan, bring the broth, bones, and onion to a boil. Lower the heat slightly. Cook at a low boil for 30 minutes.

Strain through a fine-mesh sieve, pressing down on the solids to extract as much liquid as possible. Skim the fat. Return the broth to the saucepan.

Sprinkle the gelatin over ½ cup cold water and let sit for 2 minutes. With a spatula, scrape the gelatin into the broth. Heat the broth over medium heat, stirring, until the gelatin is completely dissolved.

MAKES 5 CUPS

FISH STOCK

There is a long-held belief in French cooking that fish stock must not be cooked for more than 20 to 40 minutes. As a young cook, I ignored this rule and cooked my fish stocks for long hours, just as I did meat stocks. As I learned more, I persisted in what turned out to be a very satisfactory habit.

I eventually learned where the "don't overcook stock" rule came from. French restaurant chefs use flatfish—flounder and sole—for their stocks, because they cook these fish in quantity and have the bones and heads readily available. Also these parts, called the "frames," are often bought on their own. However, these fish do make a bitter stock if cooked for longer than 20 minutes.

If no flatfish bones are used, the stock can cook for 4 to 6 hours; this slow cooking extracts all the gelatin from the bones and makes a wonderful, rich broth. It is also better not to use oily fish like mackerel and bluefish; they make for a heavy-tasting stock. Bones and heads from white-fleshed fish like snapper, bass, and cod are preferable. I also use cod collars, the cartilage between the head and the body. These are free or very cheap. When I order a fish to be filleted, I ask for the heads and bones; I have paid for them anyhow.

5 pounds heads and bones from white-fleshed fish, like snapper, bass, or cod

Wash the fish heads and bones well to eliminate all traces of blood. Cut out the blood-rich gills with scissors.

Put the heads and bones in a pot, and cover with 10 cups water. Place over high heat and bring to a boil. Skim off the scum that rises to the top. Lower the heat and simmer the stock for 4 to 6 hours or until approximately 7 cups of broth remain, skimming as necessary.

Strain the stock through a damp-cloth-lined sieve. The stock can be used immediately, refrigerated for up to 3 days, or frozen.

MAKES 7 CUPS

VARIATION

Extra-Rich Fish Stock
Cook the broth for an extra hour to reduce it further.

MAKES 5 CUPS

VEGETABLE BROTH

For a smoother and more unctuous mouth feel, add tapioca starch to the finished broth, see the variation.

2 cloves garlic, smashed and peeled

2 medium onions, peeled and quartered

3 medium carrots, peeled and coarsely chopped

2 medium tomatoes

3 medium leeks, white part only, cut in half lengthwise, washed well, and cut across into 1-inch lengths

2 tablespoons olive oil

1 bunch spinach, stemmed, washed well, and cut across into 2-inch strips

1 cup celery leaves

Stems from 2 bunches parsley

2 bay leaves

TO MAKE ROASTED VEGETABLE BROTH: Heat the oven to 500°F with a rack in the middle.

Place the garlic, onions, carrots, tomatoes, and leeks in a large roasting pan. Add the olive oil and toss to coat. Roast for 15 minutes. Turn the vegetables and roast for 15 minutes more. Move the vegetables around in the pan and roast for 10 minutes more or until all the vegetables are nicely browned and the tomatoes are collapsing.

Place the roasted vegetables in a tall, narrow stockpot. Add the spinach, celery leaves, parsley stems, bay leaves, and 6 cups water. Place the roasting pan on top of the stove. Stir in 1 cup water. Bring to a boil, scraping up any browned bits from the sides and bottom of the pan with a wooden spoon. Pour this liquid over the vegetables in the pot.

TO MAKE PLAIN VEGETABLE BROTH: Place all the ingredients and 8 cups water in a tall, narrow stockpot.

TO FINISH USING EITHER METHOD: Bring to a boil, then reduce the heat to simmer. Cook, partially covered, for 45 minutes. Strain through a damp-cloth-lined sieve. Use immediately, refrigerate for up to 3 days, or freeze.

MAKES 8 CUPS

VARIATION

To thicken slightly, mix 5 tablespoons tapioca starch with ¾ cup cold broth. Bring the broth to a boil as described above, whisk in the tapioca mixture, and return to a boil. Remove from the stove.

GARLIC BROTH

More and more of my friends are becoming vegetarians, and in the spring, the season of good vegetables and good garlic, it is a pleasure to be able to serve them delicious soups based on a meatless stock. Garlic broth is an age-old Mediterranean staple that is cheap to make and yet offers flavor and a certain body that comes from the stickiness all of us who have peeled garlic know well.

Garlic bulbs are at their juiciest, least sharp, and least bitter in spring. When long-cooked, garlic is mild and sweet, not aggressive; even those who are put off by raw garlic's strong taste will find this broth deliciously smooth.

It is versatile, too, because it can be eaten on its own with the addition of just a few ad-hoc ingredients. Consider some jalapeño pepper, cilantro, and lime juice; diced tomato, chopped parsley, matchsticks of zucchini, and thinly sliced basil; cooked peas and small leaves of spinach; lemongrass, curry leaves, and lime juice; or anything else that appeals to you. Traditional additions, in quantities determined by the cook's imagination, are poached eggs or egg drops (for stracciatella) and thin slivers of serrano ham, or tomatoes and stale gluten-free bread, or broccoli rabe.

3 small heads garlic
1 tablespoon olive oil
Kosher salt (optional)
Freshly ground black pepper (optional)

Smash the garlic heads, separating the cloves. Smash and peel the cloves and cut in half lengthwise. If there is a green germ in the center, remove it.

In a medium saucepan, warm the oil over low heat. Stir in the garlic and cook, stirring often, for about 20 minutes or until the outside is translucent and the garlic is soft. Do not let the garlic brown.

Add 2 quarts and 1 cup water and bring to a boil. Lower the heat and simmer, uncovered, for 40 minutes. The garlic will be very tender. Strain. If using the broth on its own, season to taste. Freeze what is not being used that day.

MAKES 8 CUPS

TOMATO PURÉE

We all need this from time to time. Sterile-pack versions are quite satisfactory, but if tomatoes are in season, it seems reasonable and cheaper to make our own. This recipe can easily be multiplied by using more racks in the oven. The amount made will be used quickly. If multiplying, freeze in pint containers.

    1 pound plum tomatoes, stemmed
    1 tablespoon olive oil

Heat the oven to 500°F with a rack in the bottom third. Slick the tomatoes and small roasting pan with the oil. Roast for 20 to 25 minutes (summer tomatoes cook faster than winter tomatoes). Purée the tomatoes through a food mill using the fine disc.

MAKES 1½ CUPS

BASIC SAUTÉED MUSHROOMS

This is a technique for cooking any variety of mushrooms, from basic white button to chanterelles.

    2 tablespoons safflower oil
    ½ pound mushrooms, stemmed and cut into quarters or sixths (about 4 cups)
    Kosher salt
    Freshly ground black pepper

Heat the oil in a 10-inch skillet over high heat. When the oil shimmers, reduce the heat to low and add the mushrooms. Cook the mushrooms, stirring occasionally, until golden brown or fully cooked, 5 to 6 minutes. Season with salt and pepper to taste.

MAKES 1 CUP

MUSHROOM BASE

This base, for risotto, pasta sauce, or cooking chicken or fish, is well worth making when the mushrooms are available. The yield is enough for a risotto or pasta for at least 6 or to cook a large roasted chicken, skinned and cut into smallish pieces and poached in sauce for 6 to 8 (serve with rice).

    ⅔ cup olive oil
    1 white onion, cut into ¼-inch dice (about ¾ cup)
    ¾ pound white mushrooms, trimmed and cut into ¼-inch strips (about 4 cups)
    ½ pound lobster or other very firm mushrooms, such as king oysters, cut into ½-inch chunks (about 3 cups)
    3 cloves garlic, smashed, peeled, and minced
    5 cups chicken stock (any of the homemade stocks, pages 203–4, or sterile-pack)
    ¼ ounce dried porcini
    ½ cup Oyster Mushroom (*Pleurotus*) Base (opposite)
    ¾ cup red wine

Warm half of the olive oil in a large saucepan. Add the onion and white mushrooms. Cook over medium heat, stirring, until the onion is translucent. Add the remaining ⅓ cup olive oil and the lobster mushrooms and garlic and cook over medium-high heat until the firm mushrooms begin to brown. Soak the porcini in 1 cup of the chicken stock in the microwave for 5 minutes and strain the liquid through a cloth if gritty. Add the porcini and their stock along with the remaining 4 cups stock, the oyster mushroom base, and the red wine to the other cooked mushrooms.

MAKES ABOUT 8 CUPS

OYSTER MUSHROOM (PLEUROTUS) BASE

Since they can be grown commercially, oyster mushrooms can now be bought cultivated in a variety of colors and flavors. A spring find of wild ones on a tree is a special delight. Although I have had a bonanza of wild *Pleurotus,* I realize that many don't have such luck, so I decided to create recipes for the store-bought kind.

Serve over Soft Polenta (page 170) or use as a pasta sauce or as a soup with tender vegetables such as peas, green beans, and young carrots. To serve as a soup or to freeze, use the larger amount of stock. For a sauce, use less.

3 tablespoons olive oil

1 pound oyster mushrooms (*Pleurotus*), fibrous bottoms removed, cut along the gills into ¼-inch-wide strips (about 6 cups)

1¾ to 2½ cups chicken stock (any of the homemade stocks, pages 203–4, or sterile-pack)

Kosher salt

Put the oil in a 9-inch-wide stockpot over medium heat. Toss in the mushrooms and continue to toss while scraping the bottom of the pan. Cook until the mushrooms are reduced to a third of their original volume. Pour in 2 cups of the chicken stock and cook for 30 minutes. Add as much of the remaining stock as needed to cover the mushrooms. Do not skim.

Allow to cool. Divide among freezer containers and freeze. To use, defrost in the refrigerator. Pour off the stock and boil in a small pan until the desired quantity is reached. Add salt to taste.

MAKES 3 CUPS

TEMPURA BATTER

Many countries have battered and fried dishes, sometimes just one food such as shrimp and sometimes a hodgepodge like the Italian *fritto misto*. Tempura batter is the easiest to handle and very good but, unfortunately, last-minute. You may want to save it for an all-tempura party.

2 cups rice flour

½ teaspoon paprika

1 large egg

Just before ready to cook, place the ingredients in a medium bowl. Pour in 1 cup ice water (plus an additional 1½ tablespoons if cooking shrimp). Stir very lightly (chopsticks are good for this) so that the batter is barely combined; there should be lumps of flour in the batter and around the rim of the bowl. The batter is ready.

MAKES ENOUGH FOR ABOUT 90 PIECES, DEPENDING ON SIZE

STIFF UPPER LIP: THE STARCHES

For the gluten forbidden, wheat is the great problem. Most of us can probably abandon breakfast oatmeal and even oatmeal cookies without bursting into tears. To not eat barley will be a relief to many. The absence of wheat is a problem.

Do not "abandon hope all ye who enter here"; there is a wide variety of other starches—not just the potato—that can make the pain more bearable. While I almost always eschew the ersatz in the form of gluey bread and other soggy baked goods, I have found pastas that are more than tolerable (see page 39). They are not the rice ones unless we include Asian rice noodles, which are good particularly with seafood and in cold dishes. Beyond the pastas, a whole range of grains, seeds, and the flours made from them awaits the adventurous, and this chapter provides basic information on these seeds and grains. It also describes them, their assets and detriments, the basic ways of preparing them, and the best ways of serving them. The book's index leads to recipes using these ingredients.

America has contributed a large share of these goods. It was a continent without wheat until the arrival of the Spaniards. Besides potatoes, I have always loved polenta (cornmeal) and grits. Beans have been a major gift. I have newly fallen in love with the Peruvian quinoa. Wild rice has its place but should not be confused with rice, which is wonderful, as is buckwheat (kasha), which we can eat but should not be confused with the wheat we cannot. Then there are grains even less known to most of us; but I hope that this book will widen our horizons.

ALMONDS AND ALMOND FLOUR

Sweet almonds are the edible ones. Bitter almonds can be toxic. Sweet almonds can be used raw or roasted and are a crunchy addition to curries, stews, and salads. Blanched almonds are white, having been put in hot water and skinned.

Like most nuts, almonds can be finely ground to make a flour. It is used in baking, in addition to being a thickener.

AMARANTH

This is part of a large family. Both leaves and seeds of some species are eaten. The small beadlike brown grain with a nutty flavor is a good source of protein and certain amino acids. It needs to be cooked before eating and can be boiled, popped, toasted, or milled. *Amaranth* comes from an Aztec word meaning "not withering" or "immortal." Expect to see more of it in the future, particularly ground as an enrichment to foods. It is easy to grow and will show up in underdeveloped nations.

ARROWROOT

An edible starch, arrowroot powder is made from the rhizomes of a plant native to the West Indies. In the past, it was used a great deal, but it has been found very low in nutritional value. Its primary use is as a thickener for soups, stews, and sauces because it thickens quickly and does not cloud the food. Conversely, once it has been added to hot food as a slurry (see page 12), it can cook only for a very short time. It has one other culinary advantage that I have never tried: it prevents ice crystals from forming in frozen desserts.

BEANS

When I was in high school, I hated Latin and my Latin teacher. Nevertheless, these days I long for the clarity of Latin nomenclature for vegetables and their categories. English is more difficult because sometimes the names given to different groups of vegetables, such as beans and their relatives, are confusing. For instance, both beans and lima beans are pulses, but lima beans are not beans (despite the name). This entry covers vegetables that are true beans; other pulses and legumes are covered elsewhere in this chapter.

The number of varieties of beans available continues to grow with the popularity of heirloom varieties and curious farmers. This section is intended only as an overview of the majority of beans available in most markets today. These nutrient-rich, high-carbohydrate vegetables have always been a staple for vegetarians and vegans alike but are especially beneficial to Intolerant Gourmets, where they substitute for forbidden starches.

BEAN VARIETIES

Beans come fresh, whole or shelled; dried, shelled; and canned. The beans that can be eaten whole are all some variant of regular green beans—haricots verts, wax beans, and romano beans. Other beans are eaten shelled and sold dried, fresh, or canned. Familiar examples include black beans and kidney beans, although, as the following alphabetical list of common beans demonstrates, shelled beans are hardly limited to these two.

ADZUKI/RED BEANS: The small red adzuki beans can be eaten young in the pod but are most often shelled and dried. They are used in everything from desserts and baked goods to facial scrubs in Japan.

BLACK BEANS: Sometimes called turtle beans and most common dried, these shelled beans pair well with pork and spicy flavors. *Chinese fermented black beans* are quite salty as they are not meant to be eaten on their own. When used as a proper seasoning they add a richness of flavor not found in plain salt. Companies have started making gluten-free black bean pastas, but they are not very tasty or appealing to look at.

CANNELLINI BEANS: Commonly sold dried and especially good when cooked from this form or from fresh, although canned can be used if drained and well rinsed. These creamy white shelled beans, somewhat larger than most others, are preferred in Italy, found along with tuna in salads and as part of antipasti and in soup. Be aware that the skins of these beans tend to come loose as they cook and drift around the top of the water; just skim them off.

CHICKPEAS: See Garbanzo Beans, page 221.

CORONA BEANS: See under Lima Beans, page 225.

CRANBERRY BEANS: These are the most widely available of beans to shell that are sold fresh. Sadly, the beautiful dappled color disappears and they turn a dull lavender/purply beige when cooked.

FAVA BEANS: Favas, the only true bean of the Old World and for millennia the only type in Europe, remain a staple there and in Central America in their dried form. They used to come in their skins, but these days peeled dried favas are widely available. Mexican favas are the most common type of peeled and dried favas available today. They come both whole, with two lobes, or split, with the lobes separated. The latter cook more quickly and are good for soup, but whole beans can be used for everything else.

Fresh favas are spring vegetables in the shell. They need to be shelled and have the actual skin removed (a painstaking and time-consuming job usually reserved in restaurant kitchens for green, inexperienced cooks with limited culinary skills). When buying fresh beans, rely on your hands and eyes to pick out the best. Feel the beans to make sure they are not dried out. The shells should be plump and firm. They should also feel smooth without any soft spots. Look to see whether the seeds (inside) are bulging out, which indicates they are overripe. Look for any kind of discoloration. Try to pick beans of similar size for even cooking times.

Broad beans are small favas in their yellow shells and eaten whole. They are popular in England despite the fibrous and flabby texture when cooked.

FLAGEOLETS: These are the seeds of adult haricots verts (green beans). These pale beans are available shelled, both fresh and dried. Delicate in taste, they are generally served in France with roasted lamb and do well with the juices of meat. There are also *white flageolets*, more like a small navy bean and usually dried.

GARBANZO BEANS: See page 221.

GREEN BEANS: Eaten whole and available fresh. These grow fairly large on vines or bushes. *French green beans,* haricots verts, are thinner and rounder than regular green beans. *Wax beans* are yellow and slightly flatter than green beans. Their vibrant color makes up for their lack of flavor. *Romano beans* are also known as Italian green beans. They are flatter and wider than green beans. They can be used interchangeably with green beans in recipes using a slightly longer cooking time.

GREEN RICE BEANS: A hybrid between flageolets and white rice beans that is similar in flavor and texture to flageolets but much lighter in color. The two varieties can be used interchangeably.

KIDNEY BEANS: The common dark red shelled dried beans used in chili and to make refried beans.

MUNG BEANS: These small beans, commonly used in East and South Asian cuisines, are also known as green beans because of their green color and oval shape. They are generally eaten whole in sweet or savory preparations, as bean sprouts, or turned into a sweet paste for desserts. The starch of mung beans is used to make jellies and clear cellophane noodles. Make a note that Vietnamese spring roll wrappers are not made from mung bean starch but from rice flour, tapioca starch, water, and salt.

LIMA BEANS: See page 225.

NAVY AND OTHER SMALL WHITE BEANS: Commonly sold shelled and dried, these make wonderful soup. In southwestern France they are used for cassoulet. The most common in North America are *great Northern*.

PINTO BEANS: Pink to light red, lighter than kidney beans, these are best grown at a high altitude and eaten fresh but are also available canned and dried.

SOYBEANS: The jack of all trades of the bean world—there is almost nothing it can't do—the soybean is never consumed shell and all. On their own and fresh, soybeans are boiled in salted water for a snack or starter. These edamame can be bought precooked, although they are not as good as when you cook them yourself. Soybeans are cooked and eaten or turned into a variety of products, such as flour, tofu, oil, milk, and paste. Soybeans are also sold freeze-dried, and these make a good crunch with drinks.

Though soybeans are cooked, dried, and then turned into *flour,* it has a strong raw bean flavor and cannot be used alone. This flour absorbs much more water than other flours, is yellow in color, and tastes chalky.

Tofu, the custardlike blocks of soybean curd stored in water, can be transformed into dozens of forms. There is regular tofu and a creamier, more fragile kind called silk tofu. There is tofu ice cream, pressed tofu in brown sheets (used as a meat substitute for vegetarians), and even soft silky tofu curds used in soups and stews in Asian dishes. The uses are limitless.

Soy sauce, like wine, is available in all different varieties and vintages. Each country that produces soy sauce makes it just a little differently from others. Chinese black soy, for example, is more viscous and often sweet compared to Japanese soy. There are cheap, mass-produced varieties of soy sauce and carefully fabricated, aged-for-decades types of soy sauce. While all good-quality soy sauces are made from fermented soybeans, most today have wheat added to them. This cost-cutting ingredient is unfortunate for us Intolerants, but the good news is that wheat-free soy sauce is more widely available.

Soy milk is often used as a substitute for animal milk for those unable to digest it. This dairy-free beverage has a dairy-like creaminess but can often taste chalky. However, let the buyer beware that soybeans must usually be heavily chemically manipulated to produce soy milk, and that is why I do not drink it or use it when cooking.

Miso is the soluble fermented soybean paste that comes in several colors: white, yellow, red, and brown—the most common. The darker the color, the deeper the flavor. It is used to make soups, sauces, and, at trendier restaurants, caramel and other sweet preparations.

How to Cook Beans

BEANS	AMOUNT	COOKING TIME	YIELD	COLOR	NOTES
Cannellini	1 cup	1 hour	2½ cups	Creamy white	Tasty, great texture
Corona	1 cup	3 hours	2½ cups	Off white	Large and starchy, long cooking time
Flageolets	1 cup	30 minutes to 1 hour	Scant 3 cups	Light green	Tender with great texture
Green rice (hybrid of white rice beans and flageolets)	1 cup	30 minutes to 1 hour	Scant 3 cups	Light green	Tender with great texture, very similar to flageolet

NOTES: Two soaking methods were used. *For the cold soak method*, beans were placed in a pot, covered by at least 2 inches of water, and refrigerated overnight; to cook, beans were drained, then covered with fresh water. *For the quick soak method*, beans were placed in a pot, covered with water, and brought to a boil for 15 minutes; beans were then removed from heat, allowed to sit for 1 hour, and cooked. In both cases, beans were brought up to a boil over high heat, then heat was reduced to a simmer until beans were cooked. Some beans seemed to take less time to cook using the quick soak method, possibly because the beans begin to cook while sitting for 1 hour as opposed to those coming out of the refrigerator cold.

BEAN PRELIMINARIES

Fresh beans should be kept tightly wrapped and refrigerated, and used as soon as possible after buying or picking. They will become starchier and less sweet with time. Light will change their color. If longer storage is needed, they should be boiled briefly in heavily salted water, refreshed under cold water, and then frozen in amounts that are likely to be used at any one time.

Keep dried beans in a cool, dark, dry place in tightly sealed containers, preferably opaque. While it may seem they last forever, it is best to use dried beans as soon as possible after buying them. Older beans take longer to cook.

To prepare for cooking, wash fresh whole beans in cold running water before snapping the ends. Trim the beans by snapping off both ends (commonly referred to as "tipped and tailed").

To shorten the cooking time for dried beans, rinse them under cold running water and then soak.

Once all the prep work has been done, fresh beans may be boiled, steamed, microwaved, or sautéed. Dried beans can be soaked, baked, cooked on the stovetop, in a slow cooker, or in the microwave. Basic cooking techniques follow.

BASICS

WHOLE FRESH BEANS

BOILING: Always use water (without salt) that is at a full boil and do not cover the pot, or the beans will lose their vibrant color. Start the timer when the water returns to a boil after the beans have been added. Make sure to use a large enough pot with plenty of water so that the water returns to a boil relatively quickly. Typically, boil 2 quarts of water for every ½ pound of beans.

Whole green and wax beans, tipped and tailed—cook for 6 to 8 minutes.

Haricots verts, tipped and tailed—cook for 4 to 5 minutes.

Romanos, tipped and tailed—cook for 7 to 8 minutes.

STEAMING: Bring water to a boil. Place the trimmed beans in a single layer in a steamer basket/insert and place in the pot. Cover and cook.

Green, wax, and Romano beans—steam for 7 to 9 minutes.

Haricots verts—steam for 8 to 10 minutes.

SHELLED FRESH BEANS

BOILING: Always use water (without salt) that is at a full boil and do not cover the pot, or the beans will lose their vibrant color. Start the timer when the water returns to a boil after the beans have been added. Make sure to use a large enough pot with plenty of water so that the water returns to a boil relatively quickly. Typically, boil 2 quarts of water for every ½ pound of beans.

Cranberry beans—cook shelled beans for 20 minutes.

Favas—shelled favas take a few steps:

1. Drop beans into boiling water for 1 minute.
2. Drain and rinse under cold water.
3. Peel off the outer skin.
4. Simmer peeled beans for 5 minutes.

Soybeans—boil in the shell in salted water for 3 to 4 minutes or boil shelled for 2 to 3 minutes.

MICROWAVING: Fresh beans cook quickly in the microwave and retain their bright colors. Place trimmed beans in an even layer in a microwave-safe bowl and sprinkle them with water. Cover tightly with plastic wrap.

Green and wax beans—cook ¼ pound for 2½ minutes; cook ½ pound for 3 minutes.

Haricots verts—cook in water; ¼ pound beans in 1 cup water for 4 minutes; 1 pound beans in 3 cups water for 10 minutes.

YIELDS

GREEN BEANS AND WAX BEANS

¼ pound beans, tipped and tailed = 1¼ cups raw = 1 cup cooked

1 pound beans, tipped and tailed and cut into 1½-inch lengths = 3½ cups

3 pounds beans, tipped and tailed = 14 cups raw

HARICOTS VERTS

¼ pound beans, tipped and tailed = 1 cup raw = ¾ cup cooked

ROMANO BEANS

¾ pound beans, tipped, tailed, and cut into 2-inch lengths = 4 cups

CRANBERRY BEANS

¾ pound beans in the shell = 1 cup shelled = 1¼ cups cooked

2½ pounds beans in the shell = 1¼ pounds shelled = 4 cups raw = 5 cups cooked

FAVAS

2¾ pounds in the shell = 1 pound shelled = 3 cups raw = 9 ounces, or 1½ cups, blanched and peeled

SOYBEANS

1 pound fresh, in the pod = 4½ cups = 1 cup shelled raw = ⅔ cup cooked

DRIED BEANS

SOAKING

Cold Soak Method: Place the beans in a pot, add water to cover by 2 inches, and refrigerate overnight (refrigeration keeps them from fermenting). When ready to cook, drain the beans and cover with fresh water.

Hot Soak Method: Place the beans in a pot, add water to cover by 2 inches, and bring to a boil. Remove from the heat and let sit for 1 hour. When ready to cook, drain and cover with fresh water. Or boil for 15 minutes, drain, and cook.

Microwave Method: For 2 cups dried beans: Place in a 5-quart casserole with a tightly fitting lid. Add 2 cups water, cover, and cook for 10 minutes. Remove and let stand, covered, for 5 minutes. Uncover and add 2 cups very hot tap water. Re-cover and let stand for 1 hour. Drain. Cover with water to cook.

BOILING

Stovetop: Cover soaked and drained beans with 2 inches of water or stock. Season the liquid with herbs if desired and onions or garlic if desired. Do not add salt. Bring to a boil, reduce to a simmer, and cook until the beans are tender, 1 to 3 hours, depending on the type and age of bean. Add liquid as necessary to keep the beans covered while they cook. When the beans are tender, season with salt. Remove from the heat and let stand for 10 to 15 minutes.

Slow-cooker: Drain the soaked beans before cooking. Cover by 1 inch with cooking liquid and cook at the low heat setting for 5 to 10 hours, depending on the bean.

Microwave: Small dried beans (e.g., flageolets, white, green rice)—place 1 to 2 cups presoaked beans in 4 cups warm water in a 2-quart soufflé dish covered tightly with microwave-safe plastic wrap. Cook for 27 minutes. Remove from the oven and let rest for 30 minutes.

Large dried beans (e.g., cannellini kidney, pinto, soybeans)—place 1 cup presoaked beans in 4 cups warm water in a 2-quart soufflé dish covered tightly with microwave-safe plastic wrap. Cook for 23 minutes. Remove from the oven and let rest for 30 minutes. Cook 2 cups presoaked beans in 6 cups warm water for 30 minutes. Let rest for 30 minutes.

YIELDS

SMALL DRIED BEANS (E.G., FLAGEOLETS, WHITE, GREEN RICE)

1 cup dried = 7 ounces = 2½ cups soaked = 3 cups cooked

LARGE DRIED BEANS (E.G., CANNELLINI, CORONA, KIDNEY, PINTO, SOYBEANS)

1 cup dried = 6 to 6½ ounces = 2 cups soaked = 2½ cups cooked

BUCKWHEAT

The name "buckwheat" is misleading for many reasons. First, there is absolutely no wheat in buckwheat. Second, this distant cousin of rhubarb is not even a cereal grain but a cocoa-brown fruit. Buckwheat is nutrient-rich, containing a high proportion of all eight essential amino acids and many B vitamins. It has been used in the Middle East for millennia and is called "kasha," also the name of a dish among many Jews (see page 224). I have used it as a substitute for cracked wheat in tabbouleh (see page 28).

CHESTNUTS AND CHESTNUT FLOUR

Cooked chestnuts when glazed or coated in chocolate are a traditional treat at Christmas, but their chief season is really late fall. Chestnut flour is made by grinding dried chestnuts, and it is very popular in Italy and Austria. It is light brown, sweet, and slightly nutty in flavor, which lends itself nicely to baked goods and other sweet preparations. From a nutritional standpoint it is not a powerhouse, although it is extremely low in calories and fat compared to other nut flours. The trick to using chestnut flour when baking is to make sure there is a protein binder.

CHICKPEAS

See Garbanzo Beans (page 221).

CORN

Corn, a grass whose seeds grow on cobs that are surrounded by thin fibers called "silk" and tightly furled leaves, is the most widely grown vegetable of the Americas. Besides the many culinary uses of fresh and dried corn, it is grown as cattle feed and for conversion into alcohol both to drink and for use as a fuel. *Dent corn,* the kind intended for these purposes, is 95 percent of the corn grown.

What we eat is *sweet* or *squaw corn,* whose niblets can be yellow, white, or a mixture of the two. There is also *blue corn,* which is soft and can be made into flour. Harder varieties are known as *flint corn* and usually used for meal. There are extremely *decorative corns* that come in blue, purple, and red and generally show up at Thanksgiving in decorations. There are also special kinds of corn for popping. My favorite is *bear claw.*

Sadly, for the home-grower—like me—corn is like candy to raccoons, which seem to know just when it will be picked the next day. They strip the leaves off, eat the seeds (kernels, niblets), and neatly pile up the shucked cobs. I have given up growing it. The raccoons always win.

Corn is sweetest when just picked and becomes starchier with time. Corn can be cooked in many ways—boiled, steamed, roasted, or grilled with or without seasoning under the leaves, microwaved, or as niblets removed from the cob. Corn kernels also show up canned and frozen, which need only brief heating.

Processed corn, used to make *hominy* and flours, is made from dried kernels that are soaked in water mixed with lye and then thoroughly washed to remove any trace of lye. At this point they can be cooked and are often canned, or they are dried for further processing, usually into flour. The first grinding is known as *"grits,"* the best of which is stone-ground speckled heart (bits of black or dark brown) that retains the germ.

In order of fineness of grind, starting with coarsest, are *polenta* (yellow or white)—avoid precooked and instant—*cornmeal, corn flour,* and *cornstarch,* generally used for thickening. The most prevalent use is probably in corn flakes.

Then there is *masa harina,* used in Mexico for cooking and for making tortillas and other treats. There is also a precooked variety called "*masarepa,*" meant to be used to make Arepas (page 17). I found it less than satisfactory.

BASICS

The information that follows is for cooking sweet corn.

(page 17)

CORN ON THE COB

WASHING/CUTTING: The husks and silk protect the corn from dirt and damage. Unless roasting, microwaving, or grilling it on the cob, prepare the corn by removing the husks. Pull off the silk. Snap off any protruding stalk. If roasting or grilling whole, the husk can be used as insulation. Pull the husks back but not off and remove the silk. If desired, spread the ear with oil or seasoning. Re-cover the ear with the husks. If the grill fire is very hot, dampen the husks with water.

BOILING: Bring a large pot of water to a boil. Add the husked corn and cook for 2 to 3 minutes.

STEAMING: Place the husked corn in a covered steamer basket. Cook for 10 minutes.

MICROWAVING: Place in a single layer on a carousel or platter. Dampen the husks slightly. Cook uncovered.

1 ear	2 minutes
2 ears	5 minutes
4 ears	9 minutes
6 ears	14 minutes

GRILLING

Shucked Corn: Rub the ears lightly with vegetable oil. Grill the corn over moderately hot coals until well browned on all sides and blackened in spots, about 8 minutes.

Corn in the Husk: Soak whole ears in cold water to cover for 1 hour. Drain thoroughly and grill over moderately hot coals until the husks are blackened and the kernels are tender, about 30 minutes.

NIBLETS

This refers to the corn kernels after they are removed from the cob. The best niblets are *shoepeg*, which are white and often used in Chinese cooking. Corn kernels are also the seeds for next year's corn.

REMOVING FROM THE COB: Run a thin knife down all sides from tip to base with the knife blade against the cob. Be careful not to cut so deeply as to include part of the cob.

BOILING: Bring a pan of water to a boil. Add the kernels. Cook for 1½ to 2 minutes.

STEAMING: Place on a plate in a covered steamer basket. Cook for 4 to 5 minutes.

YIELDS

> 2 medium ears corn = 6 ounces kernels = 1 cup raw
> 1 large ear corn = 7 ounces kernels = 1¼ cups raw

CREAMED CORN

This is the pulp from the ear of corn.

REMOVING FROM THE COB: Cut through the center of each kernel by running the knife down the center of each row, splitting the kernels in half. Turn the knife over and, using the blunt edge, scrape the corn innards into a bowl. Alternatively, grate the corn against the large-hole side of a box grater. This method results in a smoother consistency but slightly less volume.

YIELDS

> 1 medium ear corn = ¼ to ⅓ cup raw creamed corn
> 1 large ear corn = ⅔ cup raw creamed corn

BABY CORN (CHINESE MINIATURE)

Ears of baby corn are not true babies but a variety of miniature corn that matures at 2 to 3 inches in length and is entirely edible. They are light and sweet with a pleasing crunch. Most of us have not cooked fresh miniature corn;

instead, we use what comes jarred. Canned baby corn has long been a staple of Chinese cooking. Fresh is increasingly available.

PREPARED

HOMINY: Processed dried corn kernels widely used in posole in the American Southwest.

COOKING GRITS: Bring 1 cup grits, 4 cups water, and 1 teaspoon kosher salt to a boil in a medium saucepan, then reduce to a simmer. Cover and cook, stirring once or twice, for 4 to 5 minutes for quick-cooking grits and 15 minutes for old-fashioned grits. Instant grits are not recommended.

YIELDS

3 tablespoons dry grits = ⅔ cup cooked

1 cup dry grits = 4 cups cooked

CORNSTARCH: 2 teaspoons cornstarch dissolved in 1½ tablespoons liquid will thicken 1 cup liquid.

POLENTA

Stovetop: For soft polenta, whisk 1 cup polenta softened in 1 cup cold water into 5 cups boiling water. Reduce the heat to simmer and cook for 30 minutes, stirring constantly. Serve immediately. For instant polenta, reduce the cooking time to 5 minutes. For firm polenta, repeat as above but whisk the polenta into 3 cups boiling water.

Microwave: For soft polenta, combine 4 cups water and ¾ cup polenta and cover tightly with plastic wrap. Cook for 12 minutes, stirring halfway through. Remove and let sit for 3 minutes. For firm polenta, combine 4 cups water and 1¼ cups polenta and cover tightly with plastic wrap. Cook for 11 minutes, stirring halfway through. Remove and let sit for 3 minutes.

Broil: Heat the broiler with a rack at the top of the oven. Slice firm polenta into the desired size pieces. Brush with olive oil and broil until crusty, about 2 minutes on each side.

YIELDS

1 cup dry polenta cooked in 5 to 6 cups water (microwave cooking requires less water) makes about 5½ cups cooked polenta

FLAX SEED

The seeds of the flax or linseed plant come in yellow or brown and contain large amounts of omega-3 fatty acids, fiber, and protein. Ground flax seed and water can be used as an egg substitute. Flax seed boiled in water creates a great binding agent for baking. See White Bread (page 17).

GARBANZO BEANS

Also known as *chickpeas*—garbanzos are the preferred term in Central and South American cooking. These pulses are usually available dried or canned but recently have been showing up fresh at farmers' markets across the country. They are extremely nutritious. Canned chickpeas are a decent substitute for those who do not have time to cook dried chickpeas (although microwaves now allow us to cook chickpeas in under 30 minutes). The plump round bean is starchy, cream colored, and delicious. Cooked chickpeas can be ground into hummus or thrown into a salad to add protein and texture. Garbanzo bean flour is dull yellow and tannish in color with great texture and high nutritional value. This flour dissolves in liquid, but because the strong bean flavor never disappears, it needs to be combined with other flours. When it is, it can be used effectively in savory and sweet preparations as a terrific binding agent.

Continued on page 224

How to Cook Grains

GRAINS	AMOUNT	WATER	COOKING TIME	YIELD	COLOR	NOTES
Corn flour (Beretta)	½ cup	3 cups	30 minutes	2½ cups	Yellow	No flavor, too firm
Cornmeal, yellow	½ cup	2 cups	4 to 5 minutes	1¾ cups	Yellow	More flavor than white meal
Cornmeal, white	½ cup	2 cups	4 to 5 minutes	2 cups	White	Least flavor. Looser than yellow meal
Grits, Bob's corn	½ cup	2 cups	5 to 6 minutes	1¾ cups	Yellow	Best tasting. Best texture
Grits, old-fashioned	½ cup	2 cups	15 minutes	1¾ cups	White	Better flavor and texture than instant
Grits, quick	½ cup	2 cups	5 minutes	1¾ cups	White	Inferior taste and texture compared with old-fashioned grits
Kasha	½ cup	1 cup	10 minutes	1¼ cups	Light brown	Good texture, slightly nutty flavor
Millet (cook covered)	½ cup	1½ cups	25 to 30 minutes	1½ cups	Yellow	Can be substituted for quinoa, although increases in size more than quinoa
Polenta, instant (Beretta)	½ cup	3 cups	5 to 6 minutes	2¾ cups	Yellow	Satisfactory in all aspects
Polenta, instant (Colavita)	½ cup	3 cups	5 minutes	2½ cups	Yellow	Satisfactory in all aspects
Quinoa (Roland) (cook covered)	½ cup	1 cup	15 minutes	1 cup	Beige	Cooks faster and is nuttier than millet
Quinoa (Shiloh) (cook covered)	½ cup	1 cup	15 minutes	1⅓ cups	Beige	Darker, fluffier, and larger than Roland grains when cooked. Tastier than Roland
Quinoa (Whole Foods) (cook covered)	½ cup	1 cup	13 to 15 minutes	1¾ cups	Beige	Lighter color, firmer texture, larger than Roland, similar in size to Shiloh. Tastiest
Rice, brown (cook covered)	½ cup	1¼ cups	40 minutes	2 cups	Dark tan	Very nutty, great texture, drier
Rice, white short grain (cook covered)	½ cup	⅞ cup	15 minutes	1½ cups	Off white	Nutty, good texture, slightly sticky
Rice, wild (cook covered)	½ cup	2 cups	50 minutes	1½ cups	Dark brown	Very nutty, long cooking time, some split grains

NOTES: Across the board, grits were more flavorful than cornmeal or corn flour, with Bob's corn grits being the clear winner in terms of taste and texture.

Not all polentas are created equal: different brands had subtle differences in cooking time, taste, and yields.

Different brands of quinoa also showed differences in size of grain, color, taste, and yields.

Wild rice took the longest to cook and occasionally split during the process. It doesn't act like the other rice because it is not true rice.

How to Use Flour

FLOUR	AMOUNT	WATER	COOKING TIME	YIELD	COLOR	NOTES
Chestnut, Italian	¼ cup	1 cup	2 minutes	⅔ cup	Cocoa	Forms skin and cracks, puddinglike, sweet, moist, and loose
Corn	¼ cup	1¼ cups	3 minutes	1 cup	Yellow	Forms skin, tasty—like corn, firm pudding texture, slightly grassy
Corn masa, instant	¼ cup	1¼ cups	2 to 3 minutes	¾ cup	Yellow	Skin forms, firmest—almost solid, tastes like corn
Flax seed	¼ cup	1 cup	5 minutes	1½ cups	Seeds in clear slime	Thick and viscous. Seeds don't dissolve but definitely make mixture thicker and starchier
Garbanzo	¼ cup	1 cup	2 minutes	¾ cup	Yellow/tan	Forms skin, tastes like garbanzo, firms up like very thick pudding
Garbanzo/ fava-bean	¼ cup	1 cup	2 minutes	¾ cup	Yellow/tan	Forms skin, tastes like raw favas, like very thick pudding
Hazelnut meal	¼ cup	¼ cup	4 minutes	¼ cup	Cocoa with dark spots	Doesn't thicken, no skin, very liquid, not soluble
Potato	¼ cup	1¼ cups	1 to 2 minutes	¾ cup	Off white	Milky looking, lumpy, pasty, salty, tastes like potato
Potato starch	¼ cup	1 cup	Instant	1 cup	Clear	Really firm, bounced back, thin skin forms, tastes like plastic
Rice, organic brown	¼ cup	1 cup	2 minutes	¾ cup	Off white	Thick, forms skin, tastes like rice
Rice, white	¼ cup	1 cup	1 minute	¾ cup	Beige	Forms skin, firm pudding texture, slightly sweet, bright white
Rice bran	¼ cup	1 cup	10 to 20 minutes	½ cup	Cloudy yellow	Rice bran does not dissolve
Sorghum, sweet white	¼ cup	1 cup	2 minutes	½ cup	Beige	Forms skin, firmer pudding texture, slightly sweet, funky aftertaste, grainy
Soy	¼ cup	1 cup	8 to 10 minutes	½ cup	Yellow	Forms thick and darker skin, cracks on surface, chalky
Tapioca	¼ cup	1 cup	Instant	¾ cup	Clear	Thick slime, extremely viscous, tastes like plastic (not recommended)
Teff	¼ cup	1 cup	2 minutes	⅝ cup	Cocoa	Forms skin, firmest—almost solid, fairly nutty, slightly funky tasting

NOTES: All findings were particularly heat- and volume-sensitive. Smaller amounts of flour and/or water were more likely to be affected by evaporation.

Cooking times were dramatically different for varying levels of heat as well.

For the above measurements, water was brought to a boil, flour was added, then heat was reduced to a simmer.

In testing involving flours, the first step was to whisk flour with cold water (subtracted from given amount), then the mixture was whisked into the boiling water.

Tapioca starch is a more ideal, neutral-tasting binding agent than rice flour, even if it tasted like plastic during testing.

BASICS

To cook 1 cup dried chickpeas:

Stovetop: Rinse and drain the chickpeas. Add to a medium saucepan with 6 to 7 cups of water. Bring to a boil, reduce to a simmer, and cook for 1 to 1½ hours (older chickpeas take longer to cook). Drain.

Microwave: Rinse and drain the chickpeas. Add to a 2-quart soufflé dish with 4 cups water. Cover tightly with plastic wrap and microwave for 25 minutes. Remove from the oven and let sit for 5 minutes. Drain.

No-Heat Method: Soak overnight in 6 to 7 cups water. Cook briefly. Makes 2½ cups cooked chickpeas.

GARBANZO-FAVA-BEAN FLOUR

Similar in texture and nutritional profile to garbanzo bean flour, but the strongest flavor here is that of raw fava beans. Must also be combined with other flours to neutralize the flavor. Great binding agent ideally used to make doughs. Also yellow in color.

HAZELNUT MEAL

Flour made from grinding hazelnuts. This meal is high in fiber, monounsaturated fats, protein, thiamine, and certain other B vitamins. The taste of hazelnut pairs well with chocolate, which makes hazelnut meal ideal for sweets and baking. It does not dissolve or thicken liquids, act as a binder, or have any other sticky characteristics. Should be used as a supplemental flour to add nutty flavor and a coarser texture.

KASHA

When the buckwheat kernel is hulled, the remaining groat is known as "kasha" in the United States. In Slavic countries, "kasha" refers to any variety of porridges made from wheat, buckwheat, rice, or oats. Kasha has both great texture and a slightly nutty flavor, making it ideal for pairing with rich meats, dried fruit, and mushrooms.

LEGUMES

A dry fruit commonly referred to as a pod. Legumes include alfalfa, clover, and peanuts. For examples of the starchy legumes known as pulses, see the entry on page 228.

LENTILS

Lentils are a type of lens-shaped pulse that are small in size but loaded with protein, iron, and other nutrients. They have been a staple for vegetarians for thousands of years. There are three main types of lentils: French/European, Egyptian/red, and yellow lentils. All varieties are dried as soon as they become ripe and are never available fresh.

The most commonly available are the brown European lentils, although the availability of the other types has improved in recent years with mail order and the legions of specialty e-commerce sites. Lentils are sold whole, split, skin on, or skin off, in a rainbow of colors including brown, green (assorted sizes), black, yellow (red inside), red, and gold.

Lentils should be stored in an airtight container for up to a year. They should be kept at room temperature until ready to cook. Lentils vary in size and composition, so cooking times will range from 10 to 50 minutes. Lentils will take longer to cook the longer they have been in storage. Do not add salt to the cooking liquid as this toughens the skins; season only once the lentils are fully cooked.

BASICS

BOILING: Bring 1 cup lentils and 3 cups water to a boil. Reduce to a simmer, cover, and cook until tender. Drain.

Brown lentils—cook for 35 to 40 minutes.

Red lentils—cook for 12 to 14 minutes.

MICROWAVE: Combine 1 cup lentils and 4 cups water in a 2½-quart soufflé dish. Cover tightly with plastic wrap. Microwave. Remove from the oven and let rest for 20 minutes. Remove the plastic wrap and drain.

Brown lentils—cook for 25 to 27 minutes.

Red lentils—cook for 7 minutes.

YIELDS

1 cup dry lentils = 2¼ cups cooked lentils

LIMA BEANS

These are not beans at all but legumes. They are one of the few things that I often use frozen (better than canned). Look for Fordhooks, named after the farm at which they were developed. Larger specimens of this variety are called "gigantes" in Greece, "coronas" in Italy, and "giant" or "extra large limas" here in the United States. Coronas, also known as runner beans or sweet runner beans, are ideal for vegetarians since they're hearty and flavorful.

BASICS

BOILING: Add shelled lima beans to boiling water. Simmer for 5 minutes, then taste; cooking times will vary with the size of the beans.

STEAMING: Place shelled beans in a covered steamer basket. Cook for 10 to 12 minutes.

YIELDS

One 10-ounce package frozen baby lima beans, defrosted = 1½ to 2 cups

MILLET

Millet is not a true grain at all but rather a grass with small, round, yellow and cream-colored kernels. It is extremely high in iron: among the starches described in this chapter, only teff has higher levels. This grass contains magnesium, phosphorus, fiber, and protein. The kernels are a delicious alternative to couscous and can be used interchangeably with quinoa. See Summer Millet Risotto, page 43.

PEAS

There are several varieties of peas, both fresh and dried. My favorites are the small to tiny peas just out of their pods in early spring. If I am lucky, I get a second crop in early fall. These green—English—peas can be climbers clinging to supports with corkscrew-like tendrils or more rarely in bushy clumps. The tendrils (shoots) can be tossed in toward the end of a stir-fry as can the small leaves.

Other peas that can be eaten fresh are sugar snaps, which are plump and eaten whole, and snow peas, which are very like sugar snaps but flat. The latter are commonly used in Asian cuisines, often cut into thin lengthwise strips. Both of these peas, which are eaten with their pods unless very young, often have strings around the outer edge that must be pulled off by breaking off one end and pulling the string slowly down both sides.

Since peas are at their best when young—they turn starchy quickly—many people prefer to use frozen peas. I have a perverse pleasure in canned tiny peas.

Most other varieties of peas are dried and then eaten only after cooking. These include black-eyed peas, a crucial ingredient of New Year's festivities in the South and the Caribbean, which are actually a bean. Split peas of a variety of colors—such as green, brown, and yellow—are commonly made into soup; in India they are often cooked, puréed, spiced, and used as dhal, a side dish.

Since a childhood disaster with dried pea soup, which I thought I had learned to make in school, I have avoided dried peas.

POLENTA

Italian cornmeal. For more information, see page 219.

POTATOES

Potatoes can be divided into groups: floury (like baking), waxy (like new and fingerlings), and colored, such as blue, which can be starchy or firm. Floury, starchy potatoes are the best to use for mashing. Waxy and firm are best for boiling and steaming. All can be fried and roasted. Oddly, some, like the golden yellow Yukon Gold, are waxy and firm when young and small and floury when old and large.

Floury potato varieties include baking, Idaho, Irish, Maine, White, and large Yukon Gold. Waxy potato varieties include California, Creamer, fingerlings, Russian Banana, and small Yukon Gold.

Potato flour cooks fairly quickly with boiling water and becomes a milky, lumpy, extremely sticky and pasty mass. It is quite salty and tastes very much like potatoes. This is an ideal starch for savory preparations in gluten-free baking and cooking where a potato flavor is desired. *Potato starch*, which is finer in texture, is used dissolved first in water and then tempered with some of the hot liquid to thicken soups and stews.

BASICS

BOILING: Wash and peel 1 pound of potatoes; cut them into ½-inch dice (about 3 cups). Add 2 tablespoons kosher salt to 2 quarts water in a large saucepan over high heat. Bring to a boil and add the potatoes. Cook until the tip of a knife easily pierces the potato.

Floury potatoes—cook for 10 to 15 minutes.
Small waxy potatoes—cook for 15 to 20 minutes.
Large waxy potatoes—cook for 25 to 30 minutes.

BOILING IN MICROWAVE: Wash and peel 1 pound of potatoes; cut them into ½-inch dice (about 3 cups). Add the potatoes to 2 cups water in a 2-quart measure. Cover tightly with plastic wrap. Cook for 13 minutes.

BAKING: Use baking potatoes that are approximately 8 ounces. Bake in a 500°F oven for 45 minutes. This produces an old-fashioned baked potato with a really crisp outer skin and fluffy inside.

BAKING IN MICROWAVE

For 7- to 8-Ounce Baking Potatoes: Prick twice with a fork. Place 1 potato in the center, arrange other potatoes spoke fashion around it; do not cover.

1 potato	Cook for 4 minutes
2 potatoes	Cook for 7½ minutes
3 potatoes	Cook for 10½ minutes
4 potatoes	Cook for 14 minutes

For Small Waxy Potatoes: Cook 1 pound potatoes with 3 tablespoons oil for 7 to 9 minutes. Or cook 1 pound potatoes in a circle on a dinner plate with 1 tablespoon water for 7 minutes.

ROASTING: Potatoes may be peeled before roasting or washed and left unpeeled. They may be slicked with olive or other oil or cooked in the fat from the meat being cooked.

Floury Potatoes: Cut potatoes weighing about 10 ounces each into wedges about ½ inch thick or into ½-inch dice. Roast in a 500°F oven. Use a small roasting pan for 1 potato (2 cups if diced), a medium roasting pan for 2 potatoes (4 cups if diced), and a large roasting pan for 3 potatoes in ½-inch-thick wedges or 4 potatoes in ½-inch dice (8 cups if diced).

For ½-inch wedges, place the potatoes in the pan and slick them with 1 to 3 tablespoons fat. Roast for 15 minutes. Turn the potatoes with a spatula, scraping along the bottom of the pan to scoop up any wedges that stick. Roast for 10 minutes more. Transfer the wedges to a plate lined with paper towels.

For ½-inch dice, place the pieces in the pan and slick with 2 to 4 tablespoons fat. Roast for 10 minutes. Turn the potatoes with a spatula, scraping along the bottom of the pan to scoop up any that stick. Roast for 10 minutes more. Transfer to a paper-towel-lined plate.

Waxy Potatoes: Cut potatoes into halves, quarters, ¼-inch slices, or ¼-inch dice. Roast in a 500°F oven:

> ¾ to 1 pound potatoes, halved (3 cups), 1 pound quartered (2¾ cups), 10 ounces in ¼-inch slices (2 cups), or 10 ounces in ¼-inch dice (1½ cups) in a small roasting pan
>
> 1¾ pounds, halved (6 cups), 1¾ pounds quartered (5½ cups), 18 to 20 ounces in ¼-inch slices (4 cups), or 2 pounds in ¼-inch dice (5 cups) in a medium roasting pan
>
> 2½ pounds potatoes halved (10 cups), 2¼ pounds quartered (9 cups), or 1¾ to 2 pounds in ¼-inch slices (7 cups) in a large roasting pan.

Roasting Whole Potatoes: Potatoes that are about 2½ ounces can be left whole and roasted in the smallest pan that holds them comfortably in a single layer. Slick the potatoes and the pan with 2 tablespoons fat. Roast for 15 minutes. Turn the potatoes with a metal spatula, scraping along the bottom of the pan to scoop up any that stick. Roast for another 15 minutes. Turn. Roast for 10 to 20 minutes more.

Roasting Halves: Slick the potatoes and the pan with 2 tablespoons fat and roast, cut side down, for 15 minutes. Turn the potatoes with a spatula, scraping along the bottom of the pan to scoop up any that stick. Roast for 15 minutes more. Transfer the halves to a paper-towel-lined plate.

Roasting Quarters: Slick the potatoes and the pan with 2 tablespoons fat. Roast, cut side down, for 15 minutes. Turn the potatoes with a spatula, scraping along the bottom of the pan to scoop up any that stick. Roast for 5 to 10 minutes more. Transfer the pieces to a paper-towel-lined plate.

Roasting Slices: Slick the potatoes and the pan with 2 tablespoons fat. Roast for 15 minutes. Turn the potatoes with a spatula, scraping along the bottom of the pan to scoop up any that stick. Roast for 5 minutes more. Transfer the pieces to a paper-towel-lined plate.

Roasting Potato Dice: Slick the potatoes and the pan with 2 tablespoons fat. Roast for 10 minutes. Turn the potatoes with a spatula, scraping along the bottom of the pan to scoop up any that stick. Roast for 10 minutes more. Transfer the pieces to a paper-towel-lined plate.

YIELDS

FLOURY POTATOES

1 small potato = 4 to 6 ounces

1 medium potato = 8 ounces

1 medium potato, cut into ½-inch cubes = 1½ cups raw = 1 cup cooked

1 medium potato = 1½ cups purée

1 large potato = 9 to 10 ounces

1 large potato, roasted = 2 to 3 servings

WAXY POTATOES

1 small potato = 3 to 4 ounces

1 medium potato = 7 to 8 ounces

1 large potato = more than 8 ounces

3 whole or halved small potatoes, roasted = 1 serving

8 to 10 quarters, roasted = 1 serving

8 slices, roasted = 1 serving

½ cup, roasted = 1 serving

PULSES

The family of legumes that includes garbanzo beans (see page 221), peas (see page 225), beans (see page 213), lima beans (see page 225), and lentils (see page 224).

QUINOA

This good-to-eat seed (grain) that came from the Andes can be served as a side or main dish or as a replacement for rice. It is a nutritional wonder with much the same protein profile as milk. It has only one problem: it is saponaceous, meaning that when put into water it foams up like suds and is disagreeable. However, most quinoa on sale has usually been prerinsed, avoiding this. If yours hasn't, remedy the situation by placing it in a fine sieve and running it under cold water.

Quinoa is one of my new favorites and can be eaten as a side dish or cooked longer to become mushy and eaten as a cereal (see page 16). It can also be used as a coating for foods that will be sautéed. There are red and brown varieties. The red is particularly attractive but takes longer to cook and never gets quite as soft as the lighter kind. Quinoa flour is also available and used for baking. For basic quinoa preparation and recipes, see page 168, as well as the table on page 222.

RICE

Rice is one of the world's most important starches and is probably eaten by more people than any other. In China and South Korea, when one wants to ask if someone has eaten, the question is "Have you had rice today?" Rice is relatively bland and, with the exception of black rice, makes a good background for other flavors, and is a fine absorber of flavors. Rice is usually polished, which removes the bran and the germ and makes it white but leaves it very low in

nutritional value. It is also ground into flour and used in batters, which become translucent when fried. Rice comes in many colors and sizes, each of which cooks somewhat differently. Different countries and different cuisines opt for different kinds of rice from that for sushi (short-grain white rice) to that for risotto (arborio, carnaroli, or vialone nano). Using a different rice will change the amount of liquid needed, the cooking time, and the result.

BASICS

Cooking times for white rice will depend on the size of the rice. Rice is stirred into boiling water, the heat reduced to simmer (if using an electric burner, move the pot to a different burner and set it to low heat to avoid residual high temperatures), the pot covered, and the rice cooked until tender.

Glutinous white rice is soaked, drained, added to water, then brought to a boil; the heat is reduced to simmer and the rice is cooked for 15 to 20 minutes.

Black, brown, red, and short-grain white rice are added to water, then brought to a boil in a small saucepan, then reduced to simmer, the pot covered, and the rice cooked until tender.

BLACK RICE/FORBIDDEN RICE

Black rice is a partially milled rice that is high in iron and fiber and has a nutty taste. Black rice may also be sold as black Japonica rice, which is actually a combination of Asian black short-grain rice and medium-grain mahogany rice. Forbidden rice is a variety of black rice so named because it was originally enjoyed only by the emperor of China in the Forbidden City. This black rice turns purple when cooked and is similar in nutrient profile to regular black rice. The rice is quite regal looking in its deep purple glory when fully cooked, but unfortunately resembles rodent droppings when raw. Nevertheless, the nutty flavor, firm texture, and glossy appearance when cooked make this rice an ideal companion to richly flavored meats like duck and pork. This sturdier grain does not get mushy in the presence of sauce or liquids.

To make black/forbidden rice, use 1 part rice to 1¾ parts water and cook for 30 minutes. The yield will be 2⅔ times the quantity of raw rice.

BROWN RICE

Brown rice is the first rice that emerges after the outer husks are removed once the rice crop has been harvested. After the remaining husks (rice bran) and germ are removed, the result is white rice. The less-processed, more-whole-grain brown rice has more nutrients, including B vitamins, fiber, iron, and magnesium, than its white counterpart but it turns rancid much faster than white rice. It is nutty in flavor, chewy, and takes much longer to cook than white rice. This rice cannot be used interchangeably with white rice when making stuffings for vegetables or meats. This sturdier grain does not get mushy in the presence of sauces or liquids.

To make brown rice, use 1 part rice to 2½ parts water and cook for 35 to 40 minutes. The yield will be 4 times the quantity of raw rice.

RED RICE

Bhutanese red rice is a semimilled medium-grain rice that retains some of the rice bran (this is what makes the rice reddish in color). The nutritional profile is similar to that of brown rice, although it takes less time to cook than brown rice and longer to cook than white rice. This rice has been a staple of the Bhutanese people and has only recently been allowed to be imported into the United States, although in limited quantities. In our testing, it was not an audience favorite. There is a slight funky aftertaste.

To make red rice, use 1 part rice to 1¾ parts water and cook for 30 minutes. The yield will be 2½ times the quantity of raw rice.

WHITE RICE

This is the polished grain that emerges once the outer husk and rice bran have been removed. Not surprisingly, there is little nutritional value left after all that processing. But what white rice lacks in nutrients it makes up for in shelf life. This type of rice can be stored for much longer than all other types of rice. There are many varieties of white rice found in different parts of the globe. The Italians have three types of short-grain white rice with a white dot in the center: arborio, carnaroli, and vialone nano. The long and slender white basmati rice is enjoyed with Indian cuisine. In East Asia, Koreans, Chinese, and Japanese enjoy short-grain white rice but prepare it with different quantities of water such that Korean and Japanese rice is stickier than the lighter, nuttier-tasting Chinese rice. In Thailand, long-grain jasmine white rice is king, while in the Americas both long-grain and short-grain rices are enjoyed. White rice has a neutral flavor, and most varieties (Italian short-grain white does not fall into this category) do not hold up well against liquids and sauces because they become soft and mushy pretty quickly.

To make long-grain/Carolina, basmati, or jasmine white rice, use 1 part rice to 1¾ parts water and cook for 15 minutes. The yield will be 3 times the quantity of raw rice.

To make short-grain white rice, use 1 part rice to 1½ parts water and cook for 15 minutes. The yield will be 3 times the quantity of raw rice. Also see the table on page 223.

GLUTINOUS WHITE RICE: Also known as sticky, waxy, pearl, botan, mochi, or sweet rice, glutinous white rice is cultivated all over Asia, showing up in Chinese, Japanese, Korean, Thai, Laotian, Vietnamese, Philippine, and Burmese dishes. A single gene mutation causes the characteristic stickiness that makes this rice different from plain white rice. Though milled sticky rice is always white, unmilled sticky rice may be black or purple in color.

To make glutinous white rice, soak 1 part rice in 3 parts warm water for 15 minutes; drain and then combine the rice with 1¼ parts water and cook for 15 to 20 minutes. The yield will be 2¼ times the quantity of raw rice.

CONVERTED RICE: Converted rice is precooked and dehydrated rice. It is a long-grain rice that takes longer to cook than other kinds of white rice. It tends to stay firmer than the others.

RISOTTO RICE: There are three types of short-grain rice that have been developed in Italy for the making of risotto. They are all short-grain and starchy and have a white, opaque dot in the middle. Arborio is the most common and white. Vialone nano, which is somewhat more delicate in taste, is also white. Carnaroli is slightly yellow and good with seafood.

To make arborio or carnaroli rice, add 1 part rice to 2 parts boiling water. Reduce to a simmer, cover, and cook for 25 minutes. The yield will be 3 times the quantity of raw rice for arborio and slightly less than 3 times for carnaroli.

To make vialone nano rice, add 1 part rice to 2 parts boiling water. Reduce to a simmer, cover, and cook for 20 to 24 minutes. The yield will be slightly less than 3 times the quantity of raw rice.

RICE BRAN

Rice bran is the husk that comes from polishing brown rice. It does not dissolve in liquid but will make it slightly cloudy. It does not behave like a traditional thickening agent, so it cannot be used in a slurry. It does not even taste very good on its own. Rice bran is a fantastic alternative to flour for food to be dredged. The bran grains themselves are quite small, so a little goes a long way. Generally, about half as much rice bran is needed for dredging food as for flour. Rice bran is loaded with vitamins B and E and fiber and is not broken down during digestion. As a result, it acts like a plumber's snake in the bloodstream, chipping away at fat deposits.

RICE FLOUR

Rice flours are made from grinding raw rice and can be made from any variety, with white rice flour being the most common. This flour is ideal for frying as it forms a very crisp crust when exposed to hot oil. Rice flour and soda water combine to make a quick and easy tempura batter. It can also be used widely in gluten-free baking. White rice flour is a relatively tasteless flour that can also be an ideal thickening agent. Brown rice flour can be used for baking and frying, although the nuttier taste and color make it far less neutral than its white sister. Glutinous or sweet rice flour is made from glutinous or sticky rice. It is also used as a thickening agent and for some desserts. When even more finely ground, it is rice starch.

For how to cook, see the table on page 223.

RICE NOODLES

Typically enjoyed in East Asian cuisines, rice noodles (also called *sticks*) come in a variety of shapes and textures. They can be translucent or opaque. The thinnest are known as *rice vermicelli* (but when made with mung bean starch they are called *bean vermicelli*) and *sai fun* (Chinese). The thinnest noodles generally come in 3-ounce bundles like skeins of wool. They often come several to a package. These noodles do not need to be cooked but need to be soaked in hot water until pliable. They can also be deep-fried in hot oil. Broader rice noodles may also be called *vermicelli* or *mai fun* (Chinese). These noodles come in 8-ounce packages and can be broken into pieces. The broadest/widest noodles which must be cooked are called *chow fun* (Chinese). The thickest rice noodles are known as *pad thai* (in Thailand) and are used in the dish of the same name. They come in 6- and 12-inch lengths. Sometimes both sizes come in the same package. To make them uniform, simply clip the longer noodles in half with kitchen scissors. The best method for these thick noodles is to soak them in water until they are flexible and then briefly cook them in boiling water.

BASICS

COOKING RICE NOODLES

Bring 6 quarts of water to a boil in a large saucepan over high heat. Add 1 package rice noodles (about 8 ounces). Cook $\frac{1}{16}$-inch-thick noodles for 3 minutes, or $\frac{1}{4}$-inch-wide flat noodles for 7 minutes. (Different thicknesses will vary proportionately in cooking time and yield.) Drain in a colander. Shock with cold running water until the noodles are cool to the touch.

YIELD

4 cups ($\frac{1}{16}$-inch-thick noodles) or 7 cups ($\frac{1}{4}$-inch-wide noodles)

VARIATION

Soak the noodles in hot water for 5 minutes, cook for 1 minute in boiling water, then finish in sauce.

For very fine rice noodles (vermicelli or sai fun), no cooking is required. Simply soak the noodles in warm water until they are pliable (depending on the noodle, this could be 3 minutes to 1 hour). One bunch of noodles equals 2 cups of limp noodles.

RICE PAPER

Rice paper is translucent, thin, and brittle. To use rice paper, it must first be soaked in warm water to rehydrate it and make it malleable. Undersoaking rice paper will result in cracks, and oversoaking will result in tears to the fragile sheets. Rice paper comes either round or square in various sizes. It can be used raw to make Vietnamese summer rolls or wrapped around filling and deep-fried.

SORGHUM

This grass is rich in iron, calcium, and potassium and is more slowly digested than many other grains, which may make it a healthful alternative both for nutritional value and as an insoluble fiber. It has a neutral color but a slightly sweet and grassy taste. When it is cooked, it is somewhat grainy, so it should be avoided in larger quantities when a smooth and silky texture is wanted.

TAPIOCA

When I was growing up, puddings made of whole tapioca were called "fish eyes and glue." The French used to use tapioca in clear soups instead of noodles. This easily digested, gluten-free starch has a limited nutritional profile in that it really provides only calories in the form of carbohydrates. It does contribute a small amount of the daily iron requirement but nothing else. Tapioca starch cannot be eaten alone as it taste likes plastic and is not recommended as a thickening agent in large amounts. The powder is white but turns clear when cooked in liquid.

TEFF

Teff is the smallest grain in the world, measuring only $\frac{1}{32}$ inch in diameter. Traditionally used to make the Ethiopian flatbread *injera*, teff flour comes from the grain of an annual grass cultivated in the horn of Africa. Teff has a favorable nutritional profile as it is both gluten-free and loaded with iron and all eight essential amino acids. It also provides calcium, protein, and dietary fiber. The grain itself has a nutty and slightly funky taste. Teff flour can be used in both savory and sweet preparations, and it can be cooked with water like a polenta to make an alternative starchy side dish. It also can be combined with chestnut flour in sweet preparations or for baking as it adds elasticity to doughs. For cooking times and recipes, see pages 169–70.

WILD RICE

Wild rice is not a true rice but a grass. It is high in protein and fiber and low in fat. It takes much longer to cook than brown and white rice. The long and slender seeds burst during cooking, revealing a bright white interior. The nutty flavor is distinct from brown rice, and the firm exterior even when fully cooked may not be enjoyed by all.

BASICS

To make wild rice, use 1 part wild rice to 4 parts water and cook for 50 minutes. The yield will be 3 times the quantity of uncooked rice. (See also the table on page 222.)

Bring water to a boil; stir in the rice and return the water to a boil; reduce the heat to simmer, cover, and cook until tender.

ACKNOWLEDGMENTS

There are many people involved in the making of any book, and this one is no exception. It was written with the help of Clara Park and Cindy Yeh, and I thank them for their contributions.

Once the manuscript was finished, two special people got involved to make it into a book. Ann Bramson, the publisher and editor in chief of Artisan, and I have worked together for as many years as my children have been adults. Her vision and passion ensure the result is a beautiful book. A new associate is Trent Duffy, the executive managing editor; he is thorough, strong, and kind—a rare combination. I thank them both.

INDEX